I0468420

# SOLVED: THE RIDDLE OF ALZHEIMER'S DISEASE

# SOLVED: THE RIDDLE OF ALZHEIMER'S DISEASE

Dr. Mark Starr MD(H)

Copyright ©2016 Dr. Mark Starr MD(H)

Printed in the United States of America.

All rights reserved. No part of this book may be reproduced in any form or by any electronic or mechanical means, including information storage and retrieval systems, without permission in writing from the publisher, except by a reviewer who may quote brief passages in a review.

Starr, Mark
Solved: The Riddle of Alzheimer's Disease

ISBN-13: 9781530509232
ISBN-10: 1530509238
Library of Congress Control Number: 2016900897
CreateSpace Independent Publishing Platform
North Charleston, South Carolina

## PUBLISHER'S NOTE:

### AN IMPORTANT CAUTION TO OUR READERS:

This book is not a medical manual and cannot take the place of personalized medical advice and treatment from a qualified physician. The reader should regularly consult a physician in matters relating to his or her health, particularly with respect to any symptoms that may require diagnosis or treatment. Although certain medical procedures and medical professionals are mentioned in this book, no endorsement, warranty or guarantee by the author is intended. Every attempt has been made to ensure that the information contained in this book is current; however, due to the fact that research is ongoing, some of the material may be invalidated by new findings. The author and publisher cannot guarantee that the information and advice in this book are safe and proper for every reader. For that reason, this book is sold without warranties or guarantees of any kind, expressed or implied, and the author and publisher disclaim any liability, loss or damage caused by the contents. If you do not wish to be bound by these cautions and conditions, you may return your copy to the publisher for a full refund.

# DEDICATION

*I dedicate this book to my wonderful parents, Ben Starr and Virginia Bliss Starr, who lived into their eighties with all of their faculties intact. I also dedicate the book to Lawrence Sonkin M.D. PhD. At age 45, my health had begun to rapidly decline and I believe his treatment to correct my hypothyroidism probably saved my life. His research has helped shed light upon the proper treatment for hypothyroidism.*

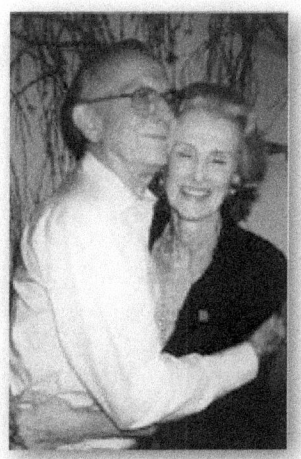

Ben and Virginia Starr

# ACKNOWLEDGEMENTS

FOR HELPING EDIT the final drafts of this book, many thanks to my dear sister, Dr. Sydney Starr, Ashton Prescott, Dr. Xan Simonson, Carol Petersen, Brenda Wilson, Dr. Ivan Danfof and Marcus Plourde. I am grateful for the research provided by Dr. David Brownstein, Dr. Jerry Tennant, and Dr. David Friedman. Their research helped cement some of the most important information contained in this book.

# TABLE OF CONTENTS

# LIST OF TABLES AND FIGURES

## TABLES

## FIGURES

# A PERSONAL MESSAGE FROM DR. STARR

## THE ARIZONA STATE BOARD OF HOMEOPATHIC AND INTEGRATED MEDICAL EXAMINERS

IT IS MY great fortune and privilege to have a MD(H) license in the state of Arizona

Arizona is one of three states that offer a medical license to medical and osteopathic physicians who meet certain criteria by passing written and oral examinations. Our board certified physicians specialize in providing integrated medical therapies and homeopathy. I am privileged to hold License No. 174, given by the Arizona Board of Homeopathic & Integrated Medical Examiners.

The Arizona Homeopathic & Integrative Medical Association (AHIMA) is the state association for physicians licensed by the Arizona Board of Homeopathic & Integrated Medical Examiners. AHIMA lobbies on behalf of the Board and provides quality education to its members.

Our Arizona homeopathic and integrated medical association (AHIMA) employs a full time lobbyist and a full time secretary. We are a small group of physicians and need all of the support we can muster.

Physicians who are licensed by the Arizona Board, like-minded professionals, and members of the public are all welcome to join and support our elite group of doctors.

To learn more about AHIMA, please visit: www.arizonahomeopathic.org

We encourage all like-minded medical and osteopathic physicians to become licensed by the Arizona Board of Homeopathic & Integrated Medical Examiners. Learn more at: www.azhomeopathbd.az.gov

AHIMA invites the readers of this book and like-minded professions to join our Association and join us in our fight to keep homeopathic and integrative medicine legal in Arizona. Join today! www.arizonahomeopathic.org

Please contact your Arizona state senators and congressmen and insist that the Homeopathic and Integrated State Medical Board be preserved for the benefit of all Americans! You can also help our cause by contributing to our organization.

— Mark Starr, M.D.(H)

# INTRODUCTION

MY FIRST SUCCESSFUL treatment to reverse early stage Alzheimer's disease was in 1996. The patient was my father.

After two years of medical study in New York, I returned to my parents' home in order to begin my first private practice.

Before I left New York to return home, my mother had told me how worried she was about my father's health. It was obvious to my mother that my dear father had begun to develop Alzheimer's disease. Dad was 82 years old at that time.

After arriving at my parents' house, it was apparent that my father's mental status was declining. His eyes had become glassy, his wonderful sense of humor had vanished, and my mother was scared to death that she was losing her husband.

While in New York, I had the great fortune to study with Lawrence S. Sonkin M.D., Ph.D., endocrinologist. He had spent his long career working at the New York Hospital-Cornell Medical Center. He wrote the first treatise regarding treatment of the menopause in 1945. He also collaborated with Dr. George Papanicolaou to develop the Pap smear.

My father, Ben Starr, was diagnosed with hypothyroidism in his mid-40s. At that time, his doctor told him he would require thyroid medication the rest of his life. However, my parents moved to Florida about 20 years later. His new physician told my father that the thyroid blood test (named TSH) indicated that he no longer needed to take his thyroid medication. My father was 59 years old at that time and had been quite healthy for his entire life.

After one year of stopping his thyroid medication, he was diagnosed with a severe case of rheumatoid arthritis. He was placed on prednisone and suffered chronic pain and mild to moderate disability for the rest of his life.

After having studied endocrinology with Dr. Sonkin, it became apparent to me that my father needed to restart his thyroid medication and to begin bio-identical testosterone. I also gave him a small dosage of DHEA (a natural adrenal steroid and precursor hormone).

Within several months, his eyes became much brighter and his sense of humor began to return. His progress continued until his mental state was relatively normal. My father's sense of humor and cognition remained intact until he died at age 86 following a botched knee replacement. The surgeon fractured my father's pelvis during the knee surgery and he died months later from a staph infection.

My mother and I were with him in their home when he died. One of the last things he said was, "What was that old Jimmy Stewart movie, Son?" I knew that he was referring to *It's a Wonderful Life*. He nodded before we told each other how much we loved each other. Shortly thereafter, his morphine drip was increased to reduce his pain and he died peacefully several hours later.

# ALZHEIMER'S DISEASE

ALZHEIMER'S DISEASE IS rapidly becoming epidemic. It is the sixth leading cause of death in America. Without a breakthrough, one in three seniors will die from this dreadful disease. Currently, the medical world claims there is no cure and it cannot be reversed.

Worldwide

According to the 2015 World Alzheimer's Report cases briskly rising:

- 10% worldwide increase since 2005.
- 46.8 million worldwide.
- Projected to double every 20 years:
  o 2030 = 74.7 million.
  o 2050 = 131.5 million.
- $818 billion in annual costs.

America

The Alzheimer's Organization of America reports the following for 2015:

- 5.3 million cases.
- 6th leading cause of death.
- $256 billion in annual costs. Projected to be $1.1 trillion by 2050.

Sources: Alzheimer's Association International Website. World Alzheimer's Report 2015 - Summary Sheet. Retrieved February 12, 2106 from: www.alz.co.uk/research/world-report-2015

Alzheimer's Association Website. 2015 Alzheimer's Disease Facts and Figures. Retrieved February 12, 2016 from: www.alz.org/facts/overview.asp

The Alzheimer's Organization of America, (ALZ.org) lists several drugs that have been approved by the FDA for the treatment of Alzheimer's. However, ALZ.org states that there is no cure.

Our country desperately needs a paradigm shift in our health care system. This shift is the only way we can realize a reversal in the tide of chronic illnesses that burden so many of our citizens.

This book will show you how to affect this shift, away from the current, failed model of heath care that is bankrupting our economy.

Of all your hormones, the thyroid is the most important! Without the crucial influence of the thyroid hormones, proper maturation and function of all the other hormone glands is not possible.

This book provides research documenting that Alzheimer's disease is due to deficiencies of our own, natural, hormones (bio-identical).

Documented research that was published in 2014 revealed that proper treatment for low thyroid (hypothyroidism) prevented heart attacks and minimized the occurrence of diabetes and all of its complications. Unfortunately, none of this information has been taught in any formal medical training.

By providing proper treatment for hypothyroidism and supplementing our own natural hormones (estradiol, progesterone, testosterone, and DHEA) we can prevent Alzheimer's disease.

# MY TRAINING BEYOND MEDICAL SCHOOL

AFTER I COMPLETED my residency training in physical medicine and reha-bilitation, I moved to New York City in order to study with and be treated by Andrew Fischer M.D., Ph.D. He was renowned for his treat-ment of soft tissue injuries (muscles, ligaments, and tendons). I saw Dr. Fischer lecture at a national conference where he presented compel-ling video evidence that showed patients recovering rapidly from their chronic pain.

I had planned on staying in New York for six weeks before taking a job at a hospital in the Midwest. However, Dr. Fischer was using tech-niques that I had not been exposed to during my eight years of formal medical training.

# MY HEALING EXPERIENCE

I HAD SUFFERED chronic low back pain for 25 years following a fractured low back while playing high school football. Dr. Fischer diagnosed that my chronic pain was not due to the old fracture. The underlying cause was from the muscle injuries that occurred during the football injury.

Dr. Fischer began treating me using trigger point injections. Doctors who perform these injections use needles to break up injured muscle tissue, which allows the muscles to heal properly. Dr. Fischer offered me a position at the Bronx Veterans Hospital and I happily accepted. I continued work with him for more than one year. This gave me the opportunity to teach Mount Sinai medical students how to perform trigger point injections and the physical therapy that is an integral part of the healing process.

Prior to moving to New York, I suspected that I was suffering from hypothyroidism. My mother and brother were already taking medication to treat the illness.

I had a number of symptoms that are frequently associated with this condition. My symptoms included constantly feeling cold, dry skin and hair, sore muscles, inability to concentrate, and increasing fatigue.

During my formal medical training, I complained to my colleagues at the University Of Missouri School Of Medicine that I was suffering from hypothyroidism. However, I was told that I was working too hard and could not possibly be suffering from hypothyroidism, because the TSH thyroid blood tests indicated I did not have the illness.

While in New York, I had the great fortune to study with Lawrence S. Sonkin M.D., Ph.D., endocrinologist. He had spent his long career working at the New York Hospital-Cornell Medical Center. He wrote the first treatise regarding treatment of the menopause, and also collaborated with Dr. George Papanicolaou to develop the Pap smear.

Dr. Sonkin was in his mid-70s when I first visited his office. He promptly diagnosed that I had hypothyroidism based upon my symptoms, physical exam, and my family history.

He shared some of his research with me that indicated the thyroid blood tests were missing millions of patients who suffered from the illness. I was one such patient.

I asked Dr. Sonkin why his research about thyroid blood tests not being accurate had not been published in mainstream medical journals.

He responded, "Because I sat in the Ivory Tower with the Maven's." Mavens are self-proclaimed experts who, in this case, used their influence to shape the practice of medicine.

In this instance the Mavens chose not to publish Dr. Sonkin's research in the endocrinology journals.

Dr. Sonkin taught me how to diagnose and treat hypothyroidism as well as how to treat women who needed hormone replacement therapy following hysterectomy or menopause. Dr. Sonkin also believed that both men and women often benefited from taking testosterone as they aged.

Unfortunately, money, power, and ego have a profound influence on the business of medicine. Health care is hands down the most profitable business on our planet. Currently, health care costs are estimated to be about 18% of America's gross domestic production (dwarfing military expenditures of 4.4%)

# ANOTHER OPPORTUNITY TO WORK WITH THE BEST OF THE BEST: DR. HANS KRAUS

WHILE STUDYING IN New York, another great teacher of mine was Dr. Hans Kraus. He was the famous pain specialist who alleviated President Kennedy's back pain using trigger point injections and exercises. Dr. Kraus worked with President Kennedy's endocrinologist, Dr. Eugene Cohen. He also worked with Dr. Sonkin for several decades. These doctors were very much aware of the integral connection between hormone problems, such as hypothyroidism and chronic pain (including headaches and migraines). Dr. Kraus was 90 years old during the time I spent with him.

Norman Marcus M.D. is a pain specialist who had coaxed Dr. Kraus out of retirement in order to learn his techniques. Doctors Kraus and Marcus always treated the affected muscles' attachments to the bones. By utilizing these treatments, most patients would successfully avoid a majority of orthopedic surgeries. Dr. Marcus and his staff of therapists alleviated almost all of my chronic pain. I am certain that the thyroid hormones Dr. Sonkin prescribed also helped to alleviate my pain.

Unfortunately, most insurance companies stopped reimbursing doctors who performed these procedures in the 1990s. As a result, very few doctors remain who perform these surgery-sparing protocols.

Dr. Marcus continues to work in Manhattan at the Norman Marcus Pain Institute. For those interested in more information regarding his muscle pain treatments, I recommend his book, *End Back Pain Forever, A Groundbreaking Approach to End Your Suffering*. His web site is: www. nmpi.com

Having worked with the best of the best, I was confident that I would have great success in my new clinic. I began my private practice in Columbia, Missouri in 1996. I specialized in physical medicine and rehabilitation, as well the treatment of muscle and joint pain. I performed all of my patients' physical therapy, in addition to trigger point injections.

After two years of hands-on treatment with all of my patients, I realized that the vast majority of my pain patients also suffered from hypothyroidism.

# LEARNING FROM THOSE WHO CAME BEFORE US: BRODA BARNES, M.D., PH.D.

ONE OF MY colleagues was aware of my keen interest regarding hypothyroidism. He gave me a book entitled, *Hypothyroidism, The Unsuspected Illness*. The author, Dr. Broda Barnes, was a famous M.D., Ph.D., endocrinologist. The book included a wealth of information and research about which I was completely unaware. It also opened my eyes to the business of medicine and profoundly changed the way that I practiced medicine.

Broda O. Barnes M.D., Ph.D. was one of the 20th century's most prolific researchers with regard to hypothyroidism. He received a master's degree in biochemistry at Case Western Reserve University in 1930, followed by a physiology Ph.D. from the University of Chicago in 1931. His mentor was Professor A.J. Carlson, one of America's pioneers in the field of physiology. He assigned Broda Barnes to study the physiology of the thyroid gland for his doctorate. At that time, the understanding of thyroid functions was in its early stages.

For the next five years, Dr. Barnes continued thyroid research while teaching endocrinology at the University of Chicago. He obtained his medical degree from Rush Medical College in 1937. The rest of his life was devoted to treating patients and conducting clinical and scientific research with regard to thyroid-related illnesses.

Dr. Barnes died in 1988 at the age of 82. His research foundation remains intact. Most of his research remains available from his foundation. (brodabarnes.org or 203-261-2101).

In 1976, Dr. Barnes estimated that 40% of all men, women, and children in America suffered from hypothyroidism. He also believed the figure would reach 50% of all Americans by 1986.

During that time, conventional medical doctors were erroneously taught that the incidence of hypothyroidism (low thyroid function) was about 5% of our population.

Having had the great fortune to train with several giants in the field of medicine, I felt compelled to follow in their footsteps.

I began writing my first book in 1998. I spent almost six years searching through historic research that had long since been relegated to the medical library archives. I found more and more vital research that had been buried or ignored. Much of this vital research is included in this book.

# THE PRIMARY CAUSE OF HEART ATTACKS IS HYPOTHYROIDISM

THE NATIONAL HEART Institute had begun a large study in 1948. It was named the Framingham Study, but was officially named, The Heart Disease Epidemiology Study. Its objective was to determine why heart attacks were rapidly reaching epidemic proportions in America.

Over 5,000 adult residents from Framingham, Massachusetts volunteered to participate in the long-term study. All were given medical exams. Those who were allowed to participate were found to be free of heart disease. Participants were examined at two-year intervals. People who later suffered heart attacks helped establish the so-called risk factors. Risk factors included high blood pressure, elevated cholesterol and having a family history of heart attacks. Men were also determined to be at higher risk of heart attacks than women. All participants were more likely to suffer a heart attack as they aged.

# DR. BRODA BARNES RESEARCH AND PARALLEL STUDY

In 1950, Dr. Barnes realized that none of his patients had suffered any heart attacks. He believed hypothyroidism was the underlying cause of the burgeoning epidemic. Dr. Barnes had learned early on that removing animals' thyroid glands resulted in accelerated atherosclerosis (hardening of the arteries). Providing thyroid hormones to these animals halted the progression of their atherosclerosis.

These animals also developed lowered immunity and suffered recurrent infections once the glands were removed. As a result, their expected life spans were halved. Dr. Barnes believed the recurrent infections that hypothyroid patients frequently suffered were the main culprit that was responsible for poor arterial health and heart attacks.

He began a long-term research study to determine if the proper treatment for hypothyroidism would prevent heart attacks. His study began in 1950 and was intended to parallel the Framingham study. His study lasted more than 20 years. 1569 patients enrolled in his study. A minimum of two years of thyroid therapy was required to be included in the study.

The average number of heart attacks in America, according to the National Heart Association study (Framingham Heart Study) indicated that Dr. Barnes' patients should have experienced 72 heart attacks. Only four patients who participated in his study suffered heart attacks, which is more than a 90% reduction in the expected number of heart attacks.

Dr. Barnes purposely did not attempt to control cholesterol, smoking, exercise, or other variables including diet. He wanted the only variable between his patients and those from the Framingham study to be the usage of thyroid hormones.

The final chapter in Dr. Barnes' book about heart attacks is named, "The Demise of the Cholesterol Theory."

Dr. Barnes explained how the cholesterol theory was founded.

# THE DEMISE OF THE CHOLESTEROL THEORY

A - THERE is a high incidence of elevated cholesterol in atherosclerotic blood vessels.

In 1858, Dr. Rudolf Virchow, "the father of modern pathology" clearly showed that cholesterol did not start the process of degeneration in the arteries. Instead, elevated cholesterol was the end product of degeneration in the arteries. This evidence has been confirmed numerous times. Additional references are available in all of my books as well as Dr. Barnes' books.

B - The second evidence incriminating cholesterol was the scarcity of heart attacks in underprivileged countries, whose populations only ate a small amount of animal products.

The autopsy studies showed atherosclerosis in the arteries of all the children who died by the age of three, in both under privileged and meat-eating countries.

Dr. Barnes' referenced one study in the Bantu population from Southern Africa in 1954. The autopsies revealed more atherosclerosis in the younger Bantu than was found in American autopsies of similar age. The Bantu only ate a small amount of animal products. It is also well established that in countries with a high incidence of infectious diseases, patients die from infections at an early age, before heart attacks can occur.

C - The third and final proof that cholesterol was not responsible for heart attacks came from Europe during World War II. Heart attacks fell precipitously during the war in European countries where cholesterol-containing foods were unavailable. Heart attacks fell as much as 75%.

Dr. Barnes reviewed over 70,000 consecutive autopsies from 1930 to 1970 in Graz, Austria. The city lay in the heart of a mountainous area that suffered endemic hypothyroidism and goiters. The Graz autopsies showed that tuberculosis (TB) had exploded during the war. People were dying from TB before heart attacks would occur.

Antibiotics and anti-tuberculin drugs were introduced to the general population at the end of WWII. This allowed people who were prone to TB and infections to live long enough to die from a heart attack, instead of TB or other infections.

The Graz autopsies revealed the incidence of heart attacks at the start of the war was 12 per 1,000 deaths. By 1945, there were only 3 deaths from heart attacks per 1,000 deaths. However, the autopsies showed that atherosclerosis in the aorta, our largest artery from the heart, had doubled in severity in autopsied patients under the age of 50. The number of patients affected with atherosclerosis under the age of 50 had also doubled. The incidence of atherosclerosis had quadrupled in only six years. The elimination of meat and dairy products appeared to greatly accelerate atherosclerosis.

Dr. Barnes' study confirmed that the low cholesterol wartime diet decreased immunity and markedly accelerated atherosclerosis

# WHY THE DROP IN HEART ATTACKS?

In 1939, PRIOR to the war, there were 27 deaths from TB per 1,000 autopsies in men between 30 and 60 years of age. In 1944, there were 55 deaths from TB per 1,000 autopsies. Deaths from other infections also rose. The deaths from TB and other infections accounted for the drop in heart attacks. The incidence of heart attacks dropped from 12 to 3 deaths per 1,000 autopsies.

Germany had a precipitous rise in TB during the war and a marked decline in heart attacks. Great Britain had a slight increase in TB and a slight decrease in heart attacks. TB and infections did not increase in America and the incidence in heart attacks did not decline.

The autopsies from 1944 and 1945 revealed severe atherosclerosis in the coronary arteries of all those who died from TB. Following the war, the incidence of heart attacks mushroomed.

What do you think the autopsies revealed in 1947 of those now dying from heart attacks? Their lungs were full of TB.

The Graz autopsies revealed only one death from heart attack per 125 deaths in 1930. By 1970, heart attacks had increased to 1 death in 14. This came about with little change in the Austrian's diet, which was similar to the American diet.

The autopsies revealed that from 1930 to 1970, deaths from infections (such as TB) had decreased by 56%. The incidence of heart attacks increased over 900% during this same time. The rate of the increase in heart attacks paralleled the drop of deaths caused by infections. Prior to the introduction of anti-tuberculin drugs in 1944, the average age of death for tuberculosis victims was 38 years. The average age of first heart attacks has remained in the 60s since becoming public enemy #1.

Dr. Barnes and the pathologist in Graz, Dr. Ratzenhofer, published their autopsy findings in the *Journal of the American Geriatric Society* in 1974. They concluded their research paper by stating,

> "It is fitting that the tuberculosis sanatoriums of the past are being converted into general hospitals for the management of heart attacks. The identical patients are being cared for, but they are arriving 25 years later with a new ailment [heart attacks]."

# MITOCHONDRIA: THE CONNECTION BETWEEN METABOLISM AND ALZHEIMER'S DISEASE

I BECAME AN alternative medical doctor in 1998 and went to many alternative medical conferences. I wanted to learn more about additional research that was not taught during my formal medical training.

One of the medical conferences that I attended was in the year 2000. The American Academy of Anti-Aging Medicine (A4M) featured a research scientist who had won the prize that year for the best research concerning Alzheimer's disease.

Dr. Suzanne de la Monte's lecture was entitled, "Oxidative Injury and Anti-oxidant Rescue of the Aging Brain." Her subject focused exclusively on a very crucial and dynamic component that is contained in every cell of our bodies. This crucial component is named mitochondria.

There are hundreds to thousands of "mitochondria" in each and every one of our trillions of cells. Most of the energy production in our bodies is produced by the mitochondria. They are the main focus of research in many biochemistry departments. A growing number of medical meetings and conferences are devoted entirely to the study of mitochondria. Several journals are exclusively devoted to the subject.

Dr. de la Monte stated that for Alzheimer's patients:

- The energy metabolism in the mitochondria was decreased.
- The amount of enzyme formation in Alzheimer's' patients was also decreased.
- The number of mitochondria is decreased.
- Females are affected more than males.
- The incidence is much higher in developed nations with lower early death rates.
- The incidence increases with age.

I was unaware until that time of the connection between the mitochondria and our metabolism. However, I was aware that the thyroid gland controlled our body's metabolism and wondered how the thyroid and mitochondria were connected.

Thyroid hormones both stimulate the cellular energy production necessary for life, as well as maintaining our bodies' relatively constant temperature. The thyroid orchestrates the development of our brain and sexual maturation. Its hormones stimulate synthesis of the protein building blocks that are necessary for normal growth and to replenish the constant turnover of billions of cells that keep us healthy and renew our bodies.

Harmful cellular waste products accumulate without proper thyroid function. The immune system is dynamic, energy intensive, and dependent upon normal thyroid function. No matter what you eat or how much you exercise, your health will suffer without proper thyroid function.

Following her lecture, I was anxious to find a connection between the mitochondria and our thyroid hormones. I was elated to find the following statement in *The Textbook of Medical Physiology*:

"It seems almost to be an obvious deduction that the principal function of thyroxin [thyroid hormone] might be simply to increase the number and activity of mitochondria."

It appears to me that this simple fact has been overlooked by the vast majority of research scientists who have been focusing all their research on the mitochondria. They are unable to see the forest for the trees. The following synopsis illuminates my point regarding the connection between mitochondria, hypothyroidism, and Alzheimer's disease.

According to Dr. de la Monte:

A.  Energy metabolism is decreased in the mitochondria. I knew decreased energy metabolism was a hallmark of hypothyroidism. Many patients who suffer from hypothyroidism are always cold, because their thyroid is not producing enough thyroid hormones to supply the energy to keep them warm.

B.  The amount of enzyme formation in these patients' mitochondria is also decreased. I have listed all of the known physiological functions attributed to our thyroid hormones in each of my books' appendices (see Appendix C). These functions include: thyroid hormones increase the transcription of large numbers of genes. Therefore, in virtually all cells of the body, great numbers of proteins and other substances are synthesized. The net result is an increase in functional activity throughout the body.

Thyroid hormones activate nuclear receptors and initiate the transcription process. Then large numbers of different types of messenger RNA* are formed. Within a few minutes or hours, RNA translation on the cytoplasmic ribosomes form hundreds of new intracellular proteins.

*Messenger RNA molecules convey genetic information from the DNA to the ribosomes, where they specify the amino acid sequence of the protein products.*

It is believed that most, if not all, of the actions of thyroid hormones result from the subsequent enzymatic and other functions of these new proteins.

In other words, the amount of enzyme formation is dramatically increased in every cell of the body, including the mitochondria, when proper treatment of thyroid is administered.

C. Females are affected more than males. This is one more hallmark of hypothyroidism. Virtually, all physicians are aware that women suffer hypothyroidism more frequently than men. In addition, women are often more severely affected from their hypothyroidism. The American Thyroid Association states that women are five to eight times more likely than men to have thyroid problems.

Alzheimer's disease is also much more pervasive in women. In America the ratio is 2 women to 1 man.

D. The number of mitochondria is decreased in those with Alzheimer's disease. Thyroid hormones increase the size and number of mitochondria.

E. The incidence is much higher in developed nations with lower early death rates.

One of the hallmarks of hypothyroidism is susceptibility to infection. **Dr. Barnes' research indicated that all of the** *children who died before the age of three had evidence of prior infection in their arteries.* Developed nations provide much greater health care for their citizens, which permit their populace to receive antibiotics and other health care. This care allows the populace to survive much longer, despite suffering from hypothyroidism for much of their lives. Many more people were able to live into their 60s, which is the average age when heart attacks begin to frequently occur.

When I lecture about hypothyroidism and Alzheimer's disease, I teach my audience that everything I am going to say about hypothyroidism also pertains to the mitochondria.

Dr. Douglas Wallace was with first to publish extensive research regarding mitochondrial in the *Scientific American* in 1997. His research showed that people born with mitochondrial deficiencies often become ill only after a period of decades and their conditions usually worsen over time. Mothers with severe mitochondrial deficiencies tend to have more severely affected children. Common symptoms include heart failure, diabetes, kidney problems, diseases related to aging, neurological and muscular problems, and Alzheimer's Disease.

All of these medical problems were extremely rare in the patients who participated in Dr. Barnes' heart attack study. I have followed Dr. Barnes's protocols for the treatment of hypothyroidism for the last 18 years. My patients (over 1,500 patients in 18 years) fared just as well as Dr. Barnes' patients.

More specific documentation is in my book, *How to Prevent Heart Attacks, Heart Failure, and Diabetes.*None of my patients who have reached a therapeutic dosage of thyroid hormones have suffered from Alzheimer's disease or dementia, unless they already were suffering from the illness before they first sought my help.

Mitochondria are responsible for converting energy from the food you ingest into usable "currency."

Carbohydrates, fats, and proteins are broken down inside your cells into components that enter the cellular powerhouses known as mitochondria. Throughout this cellular journey, these "macronutrients" undergo a complex series of biochemical transformations that generate adenosine triphosphate (ATP), the molecular energy currency behind all biological functions. To give you an idea of ATP's life-sustaining importance, your body converts a volume of ATP equal to your entire weight every day. This energy-intensive process throws off an immense number of electrons within the mitochondria, resulting in constant exposure to free radicals—and rendering the mitochondria especially vulnerable to oxidative damage.

The result is a cellular death spiral: the mitochondria gradually deteriorate, leading to a decrease in vital ATP production and a deadly increase in free radical generation. Over time, this continuous free-radical onslaught destroys the mitochondria through progressive membrane damage and molecular decay. As levels of oxidative damage from mitochondrial dysfunction steadily rise with age, the body's antioxidant defenses gradually weaken at the same time, accelerating cellular senescence and death.

Left unchecked, this fatal cycle speeds the general decline in overall function that accompanies aging and contributes to the onset of degenerative disease.

CoQ10's rejuvenating power Coenzyme Q10 (CoQ10) powerfully safeguards mitochondria from age-related decay and death through two principal pathways.

Dense with mitochondria, the heart requires more energy than any other organ—and the greatest concentration of CoQ10. This is especially true for aging individuals, even those with advanced chronic heart disease. CoQ10 levels in our vital organs, like the heart, steadily rise after birth and peak at about 20 years of age.

After that, they undergo a continuous decline.18 Fortunately, three decades of cutting-edge research have shown us how to restore CoQ10 levels in the mitochondria to slow and even reverse the effects of aging.

In pre-clinical models, CoQ10 supplementation protects tissue from lethal DNA damage and increases lifespan. It boosts mitochondrial function and total energy output in heart muscle in aging animals. And in animal models, lifelong CoQ10 supplementation has been shown to decrease oxidative damage in skeletal muscle, increase native antioxidant enzymes, and favorably modify age-related changes in muscular energy metabolism.

Until 2007, the only form of CoQ10 available was ubiquinone. Unfortunately, the ubiquinone formofCoQ10 has limited absorption. Another form of CoQ10, known as ubiquinol, remains up to eight times longer in the blood. Supplementation with CoQ10 and other antioxidants and heart-energizing nutrients such as L-carnitine and taurine reduces distended heart volume in patients—a vital factor in reducing the risk of bypass surgery. Following a heart attack, cardiac tissue is at great risk for further injury, including a second attack. In patients recovering from recent heart attacks, just 120 mg of CoQ10 per day produced remarkable benefits. Supplemented patients also had increased high-density lipoprotein (HDL) and dramatically lower measures of oxidative stress.

CoQ10 also benefits people undergoing cardiac surgery, particularly older adults whose outcomes tend to be worse than younger people's, owing to declining mitochondrial function and density in heart tissue. Mitochondria are the cellular organelles that power every energy-requiring bodily process.  •  Progressive loss of function in the mitochondria—the cellular power generators responsible for nearly all energy output in the body—speeds cell aging and death.

A handful of mitochondrial-energizing nutrients have been shown to offer powerful protection from mitochondrial damage and dysfunction. CoQ10 speeds mitochondrial electron transport, increases energy production, and protects tissues from mitochondrial decline.  •  Shilajit, an ancient Indian adaptogen, enhances CoQ10's mitochondrial benefits and supports levels of the active ubiquinol form. R-alpha-lipoic acid further supports mitochondrial energy production.  •  Acetyl-L-carnitine "feeds" energy-releasing molecules to mitochondria, improving their efficiency and preventing and moreover, reversing cellular damage

# A DEVASTATING MANDATE!

IN THE 1970s, almost all of the doctors in the western world were instructed to begin using a thyroid blood test named the Thyroid Stimulating Hormone (TSH). Doctors were told that this blood test should determine whether or not a patient suffered from hypothyroidism.

*This mandate is largely responsible for our plaque of chronic illnesses, including heart disease, Diabetes, and Alzheimer's Disease.* In patients who are diagnosed with hypothyroidism, doctors have been taught to prescribe just enough of the thyroid hormones in order to normalize the TSH blood test results. These "normal values" have continued to fluctuate.

Ever since this mandate, patients have been told that they cannot have hypothyroidism because their blood test is in the normal range. In spite of having numerous symptoms associated with hypothyroidism, doctors are taught to ignore all of the known symptoms in favor of using only the TSH results. Complete reliance on the TSH blood test has led to tragic consequences for millions of people.

A significant number of doctors have been sanctioned by their medical boards for not following this mandate. When I lectured in Sweden, I learned that the Swedish doctors were forced to use only the TSH to diagnose the illness. They were also forced to use the synthetic thyroid hormone (Levothyroxin) to treat their patients.

There was a progressive group of patients who tried to change the mandate in Sweden but failed to do so. (The group posted the figure of Christ on a cross with the TSH underneath the cross.) I have also tried to help other progressive groups in Scotland and Finland to no avail.

A growing number of American web sites are attempting to bring attention to the TSH debacle. (www.stopthe thyroid madness.com, www. thyroid.about.com, www.hypothyroidmom.com, and www.mercola. com are several of the more popular sites.

Treating thyroid blood tests instead of patients' symptoms has resulted in a decrease by more than half of the dosages that were formerly prescribed since the first cure in the late nineteenth century The current dosages of thyroid hormones that are routinely prescribed for the vast majority of hypothyroid patients are insufficient to stop heart attacks, diabetes, and Alzheimer's disease.

The first medical journal to publish before and after treatment photographs that documented cures for hypothyroidism was published in 1915.

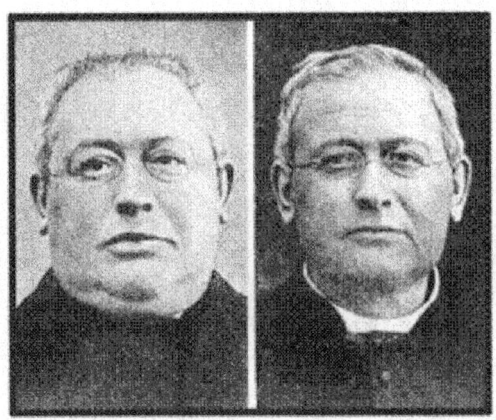

Before Treatment      After Treatment

Hertoghe, E., *The Practitioner*, Vol XCIV, No1, Jan1915, 26-69

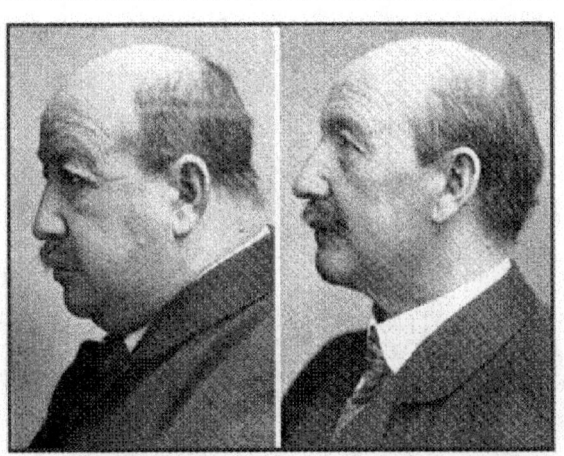

Before Treatment      After Treatment

Hertoghe, E., *The Practitioner*, Vol XCIV, No1, Jan1915, 26-69

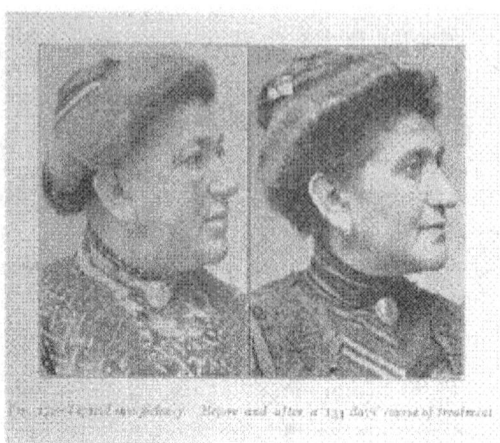

Before Treatment       After Treatment

Hertoghe, E., *The Practitioner*, Vol XCIV, No1, Jan1915, 26-69

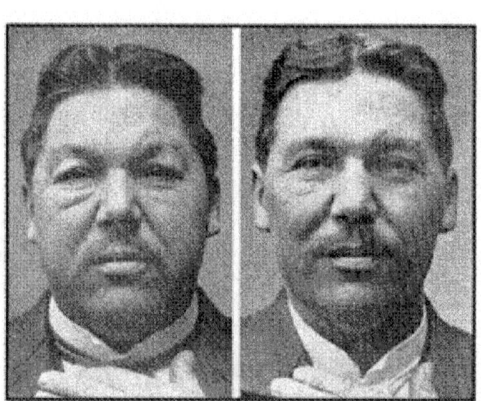

Before Treatment       After Treatment

Hertoghe, E., *The Practitioner*, Vol XCIV, No1, Jan1915, 26-69

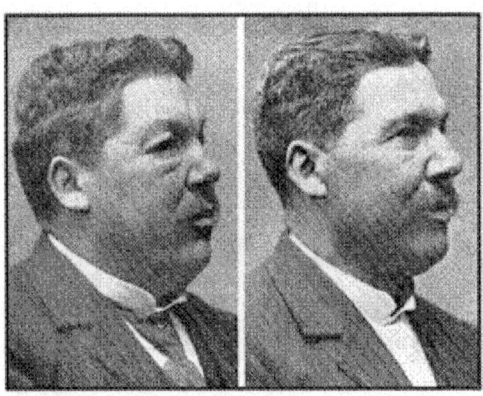

Before Treatment          After Treatment

Hertoghe, E., *The Practitioner*, Vol XCIV, No 1, Jan 1915, 26-69

Lisser, H., Escamilla, R; Atlas of Clinical Endocrinology, C.V. Mosby Company 1957

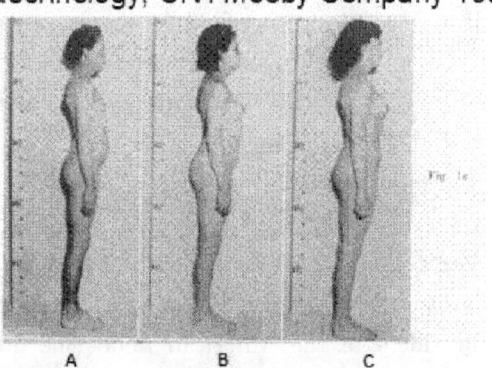

A          B          C

A. Patient's profile, no hair on arms or legs, height 4 feet 11 inches (150 cm), absence of pubic hair.
B. After 10 months of thyroid breasts enlarge, about to be married.
C. 13 months later, 2 grains thyroid, 1 mg estrogen, breasts and pelvis enlarged further, libido increased, increased height.

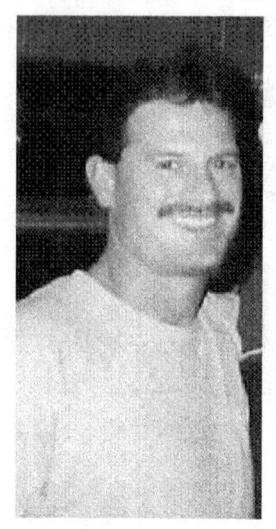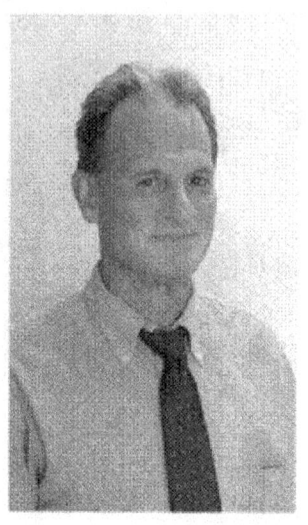

*Dr. Starr at age 40 years old (when symptomatic) and again 7 years later after 3 years of thyroid therapy.*

The original medical term for hypothyroidism was named myxedema." Myx" is the Greek word for mucin. Mucin is a normal constituent of all our tissues. It is a jelly-like material that spontaneously accumulates in about half of all people that are suffering from hypothyroidism. Edema means swelling. The following pictures will illustrate the profound physiological changes that occur in hypothyroid patients after proper treatment for their hypothyroidism.

The last medical textbook that contained "before and after treatment" photographs was published in 1957. Its distinguished authors were Dr. Lisser, President of the American Endocrine Society, and Dr. Escamilla, both whom spent their careers at the University of California Endocrinology Clinic in San Fransisco.

The following photographs with case study are from Dr. Escamilla's and Dr. Lisser's 1957 textbook. They represent a remarkable illustration of how wrong the traditional treatment of hypothyroidism has become.

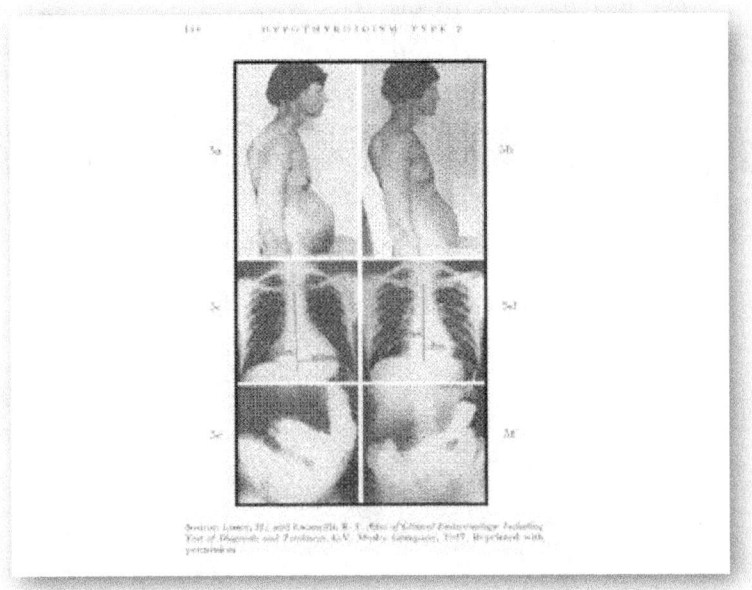

This 45 year old woman complained of weakness, sore and stiff joints, slowing of mental and physical activity, impairment of memory, slowing of speech, dryness of skin, lack of perspiration, cold intolerance, loss of eyebrows and body hair, increasing constipation and heavy periods. She also had an accumulation of fluid in her abdominal cavity (ascites), yellowish skin (carotinemia), an enlarged heart and a basal metabolism rate that was 41% below normal. The patient's appearance before and after three months of therapy demonstrates resolution of the abdominal fluid (ascites), normalization of heart size, and markedly improved tone in her colon. Her periods normalized and her heart rate increased from 51 beats per minute to 84. The doctors named her form of hypothyroidism "Internal Myxedema." Drs. Lisser and Escamilla treated her initially with 2 grains of dessicated thyroid and slowly increased the dosage to 4 grains daily. I have included this case study from their textbook to verify that these wonderful doctors prescribed 4 grains of desiccated thyroid, which enabled her complete recovery.

After 3 months of proper treatment using desiccated thyroid (Beginning at 2 grains and increased slowly to 4 grains a day), her symptoms were resolved.

# PROPER DOSAGES FOR TREATING HYPOTHYROIDISM

FIRST, THE THYROID blood tests fail to diagnose a large percentage of patients who suffer from hypothyroidism. Second, desiccated thyroid is more efficacious than the synthetic thyroid hormones.

For the first half of the 20<sup>th</sup> century, the only form of thyroid that was commercially available was desiccated (dried) porcine (pig) thyroid glands that were processed by the Armour Meat Packing Company. The dosages prescribed were measured in grains. One grain is approximately 65 milligrams.

Armour thyroid was the only preparation used in Dr. Barnes' study. The dosages that were prescribed to the study participants ranged from 2 grains (approximately 130 mg) to a maximum of 5 grains. The average adult dosage was between 3 grains and 3 ½ grains in Dr. Barnes' study. All four patients who suffered heart attacks during his study were on the minimum dosage of two grains. Dr. Barnes thought that his patients might not have suffered any heart attacks, if he had he slightly raised the minimum dosage.

For the last 18 years, I have prescribed more than two grains for all of my adult patients. My patients average dosages were the same as Dr. Barnes's patients. (3 to 3 ½ grains.) Only one of my patients taking more than 2 grains suffered a heart attack. This patient had four stints

DR. MARK STARR MD(H)

in his coronary arteries before he became a patient of mine. Dr. Barnes stated the bigger the beast, the bigger the Bullit (dosage). All of the morbidly obese adult patients that I have treated have required at least 5 grains daily in order to recover their health.

I purchased Dr. Barnes' recorded lectures from his research foundation. The lectures were recorded during the 1970s, when he was in his 70s. The lectures lasted more than two hours. They summarized much of his life's work.

Near the end of his lecture, Dr. Barnes accepted questions from his audience of doctors. One of the doctors asked him if his patients' ever died. This doctor obviously doubted

Dr. Barnes stated that almost all of the patients in his research study were living into their 80s and 90s with all their faculties intact.

I never forgot the fact that his patients taking liberal amounts of desiccated thyroid hormones did not suffer any serious cognitive problems.

# DR. EDWARD FRIEDMAN'S CRUCIAL RESEARCH ABOUT PREVENTION OF ALZHEIMER'S DISEASE

A RESEARCH SCIENTIST from the University of Chicago, Dr. Edward Friedman, performed groundbreaking research involving bio-identical hormones and their relation to Alzheimer's disease and cancer. Discovering his research provided the impetus for me to write this book.

Dr. Friedman's findings showed that our natural hormones (bio-identical) including testosterone, estradiol, progesterone, and Vitamin D were able to help prevent Alzheimer's disease. His book, *The New Testosterone Treatment: How You and Your Doctor Can Fight Breast Cancer, Prostate Cancer, and Alzheimer's* is a must read for all doctors who are interested in preventing Alzheimer's disease and cancer.

Dr. Friedman did not investigate the thyroid hormones' ability to prevent Alzheimer's disease.

According to Dr. Friedman, only the real thing will work. "The hormone receptor is everything and only bio-identical hormone structures will fit into the receptor correctly."

He stated that given the evidence of the remarkable interplay of hormones in the known problems associated with Alzheimer's, and the lack of any other effective treatment developed thus far, shouldn't keeping hormones at optimal levels in the brain be a priority for us?

He describes how bio-identical hormones help prevent Alzheimer's disease in nine different and documented ways.

# ALZHEIMER'S PREVENTION

TWO ABNORMALITIES COMMONLY associated with Alzheimer's are beta amyloid plaques between neurons in the brain and neurofibrillary tangles within the neurons. The tangles are composed of hyperphosphorylated tau protein, which eventually kills the neuron. Impaired glucose metabolism in the brain and poor blood circulation to the brain are associated with Alzheimer's. Alzheimer's disease destroys brain function and is ultimately fatal.

Alzheimer's disease has received significant attention by the medical world because it accounts for the majority of dementia cases (Katzman, 2008). In an attempt to unravel the mysteries of AD etiology and progression, some researchers sought to find an association with prior or concurrent medication use. Past research has focused on relationships between dementias and a broad spectrum of drug classes, including estrogens (Slooter et al., 1999), antidepressants (Mayeux and Sano, 1999), anti-hypertensives (Yasar et al., 2006), and statins (Hayden et al., 2005). However, a void exists regarding thyroid hormone supplementation. Our study attempts to help fill this research void by examining possible associations between use of thyroid medications and Alzheimer's onset.

Generally patients who report either ongoing or previous thyroid dysfunction at the baseline assessment were identified in 80% of contemporary studies to have atleast minor, premature cognitive impairment.

This was the sole criteria for defining and identifying thyroid disease as information concerning serum thyroid hormone levels. Use of thyroid hormone replacement therapy at the baseline assessment was ascertained, and was defined as any form of exogenous T3 or T4 and included all forms of levothyroxine and liothyronine of both synthetic and natural origin..

The hypothesis that higher levels of bioavailable testosterone, but not of bioavailable estradiol, are associated with better cognitive function in older men. In addition, bioavailable measures of testosterone may better reflect hormone levels available to the brain and thus be more closely associated with central nervous system outcomes such as cognition. Future studies, especially randomized trials, should be undertaken to determine whether testosterone may protect against cognitive decline in older men.

J Am Geriatr Soc 50:707– 712, 2002.

Several recent studies suggest that estrogen may improve cognitive function in older women and decrease the risk of developing cognitive disorders such as Alzheimer's disease. Androgen receptors tend to co-localize with estrogen receptors in the rodent brain and are distributed in areas critical for learning and memory, such as the thalamus, the hippocampus, and the deep layers of the cerebral cortex. Testosterone is converted to estrogens by aromatase, which are present throughout the body, including the central nervous system. Thus, testosterone could exert an effect on cognition in men independently or indirectly via conversion to estrogens. Although several studies in young men have examined the correlation of serum levels of testosterone and cognitive function, especially visuospatial abilities, very few studies have been conducted on older men. Recently, Barret-Connor et al. found that, in 547 older men, high serum bioavailable testosterone levels were associated with better performance on two of 12 cognitive tests administered. However, cognitive testing was conducted approximately 5 years after the hormones were measured.

Another recent study in 2014, found that testosterone supplementation improved working memory in 19 older men and that this improvement was positively associated with serum free testosterone level but negatively associated with serum total estradiol level. Emerging data indicate that growth hormone(GH) therapy could have a role in improving cognitive function. GH replacement therapy in experimental animals and human patients counteracts the dysfunction of many behaviors related to the central nervous system (CNS). Various behaviors, such as cognitive behaviors related to learning and memory, are known to be induced by GH; the hormone might interact with specific receptors located in areas of the CNS that are associated with the functional anatomy of these behaviors.

GH is believed to affect excitatory circuits involved in synaptic plasticity, which alters cognitive capacity. GH also has a protective effect on the CNS, as indicated by its beneficial effects in patients with spinal cord injury. Data collected from animal models indicates that GH might also stimulate neurogenesis. This Review discusses the mechanisms underlying the interactions between GH and the CNS, and the data emerging from animal and human studies on the relationship between GH and cognitive function. In this article, particular emphasis is given to the role of GH as a treatment for patients with cognitive impairment resulting from deficiency of the hormone. Essential Fatty Acids and the Brain.

According to research at the University of Bristol, the amount of fatty acids in the brain varies between healthy people and those with Alzheimer's Disease These findings, published in the journal

Neurochemical Research, will help researchers understand what's happening in the brain during the disease.

Seth Love, Professor of Neuropathology at the Univ. of Bristol, who led the work, says: "Fatty acids are essential to the way our brains work; they affect the way nerve cells function and help insulate the electrical signals that transmit information around our brains. When we compared the brains of people without Alzheimer's to those with the disease, we found a reduction in two types of fatty acid, and an increase in two others. It might be that the changes in amounts of fatty acids contribute to the development of Alzheimer's disease, or are a consequence. We need to do more research to find out."

Rebecca Wood, CEO of the Alzheimer's Research Trust, says: "Dementia research in Bristol is making fantastic progress. It's vital that we understand the changes in the brain that cause Alzheimer's so that we can open the door to new treatments and ways to prevent the disease. "We don't know if taking fatty acid supplements or altering our diets could have any effect on Alzheimer's risk, but this new research is helping us to understand how fatty acids might be involved in the disease," says Wood. "Over 4,300 people in Bristol have dementia, a number forecast to rise as the population ages.

We must invest in research now to find ways to prevent, treat or cure this devastating disease." Omega-3 fatty acids are considered essential fatty acids. They are necessary for human health, but the body can't make them. You have to get them through food. Omega-3 fatty acids are found in fish, such as salmon, tuna, and halibut, other seafood including algae and krill, some plants, and nut oils. Also known as polyunsaturated fatty acids (PUFAs), omega-3 fatty acids play a crucial role in brain function, as well as, normal growth and development. They have also become popular because they may reduce the risk of heart disease. The American Heart Association (AHA) recommends eating fish (particularly fatty fish such as mackerel, lake trout, herring, sardines, albacore tuna, and salmon) at least 2 times a week.

Research shows that omega-3 fatty acids reduce inflammation and may help lower risk of chronic diseases such as heart disease, cancer, and arthritis. Omega-3 fatty acids are highly concentrated in the brain and appear to be important for cognitive (brain memory and performance) and behavioral function. In fact, infants who do not get enough omega-3 fatty acids from their mothers during pregnancy are at risk for developing vision and nerve problems. Symptoms of omega-3 fatty acid deficiency include fatigue, poor memory, dry skin, heart problems, mood swings or depression, and poor circulation.

It is important to have the proper ratio of omega-3 and omega-6 (another essential fatty acid) in the diet. Omega-3 fatty acids help reduce inflammation, and most omega-6 fatty acids tend to promote inflammation. The typical American diet contains 14 to 25 times more omega-6 fatty acids than omega-3 fatty acids, which many nutritionally- oriented physicians consider to be way too high on the omega-6 side. Indeed, studies suggest that higher dietary omega-6 to omega-3 ratios appear to be associated with worsening inflammation over time and a higher risk of death among hemodialysis patients.

The Mediterranean diet, on the other hand, has a healthier balance between omega-3 and omega-6 fatty acids. Many studies have shown that people who follow this diet are less likely to develop heart disease. The Mediterranean diet emphasizes foods that are rich in omega-3 fatty acids, including whole grains, fresh fruits and vegetables, fish, olive oil, garlic, and moderate wine consumption.

Progressive loss of function in the mitochondria—the cellular generators responsible for nearly all the body's energy output—speeds aging and death. tochondrial dysfunction has been linked to an array of degenerative illnesses, ranging from diabetes and neurological disorders to heart failure. In 2007, a group of researchers reported a major (but little-known) breakthrough in our understanding of how mitochondrial dysfunction unfolds—and what can be done to protect yourself against its lethal impact.

They discovered that potentially deadly defects in human mitochondria, including molecular decay and membrane injury, begin to appear and can be detected nearly a decade before the onset of permanent damage to the DNA.

More importantly, their analysis revealed that in its initial stages, mitochondrial dysfunction is reversible, enabling the life and health of cells to be prolonged at the molecular level. The key lies in early interventions to ensure optimal mitochondrial function before irreversible DNA damage occurs. In this article, we review the latest research on a set of compounds that specifically target and enhance mitochondrial function through multiple modes of action.

# NINE WAYS HORMONES HELP PREVENT ALZHEIMER'S DISEASE:

1. Apolipoprotein Ee4 is a genetic mutation, which hinders beta amyloid excretion from the brain. Vitamin D3 increases the excretion of beta amyloid from the brain.
2. Beta amyloid secretion is impaired by both testosterone and estradiol. Cycling with progesterone also enhances this impairment ability of estradiol.
3. Beta amyloid is a peptide created from 40 or 42 amino acids. An increased ratio of the 42 amino acid structure over the 40 is associated with Alzheimer's. This ratio is decreased by testosterone.
4. Alpha secretase is an enzyme that prevents production of beta amyloid. Both estradiol and testosterone increase alpha secretase activity.
5. Beta secretase is an enzyme that increases the production of beta amyloid. Estradiol and testosterone decrease beta secretase.
6. The enzyme neprilysin degrades beta amyloid. Testosterone and estradiol increase neprilysin activity.
7. The hyperphosphorylation of tau protein is inhibited by testosterone but not by estradiol. However, progesterone also inhibits it!
8. Both estradiol and testosterone improve brain cell glucose metabolism.

9. The impaired blood flow to the brain also demonstrated in Alzheimer's disease is improved by both testosterone and estradiol.

Dr. Friedman's research helps solidify the fact that a lack of our own hormones is the root cause of numerous chronic illnesses, including Alzheimer's disease.

**Bio-identical hormones are the most powerful medicines known to mankind.**

It is quite fitting that Dr. Barnes obtained his Ph.D. in physiology of the thyroid gland at the University of Chicago in 1930. Dr. Friedman's research at the same university has provided the final exclamation point on Dr. Barnes' lifetime of work, more than 80 years later.

Estrogens are one of the best-studied classes of molecules for their potential role as a preventative or a disease-modifying therapy for Alzheimer's disease (AD). These polyphenols have been extensively assessed for their capacity to protect neurons from a number of toxic insults, including $A\beta$ peptide; in animal models of Alzheimer's neuropathology; and in epidemiological assessments given the hundreds of millions of women years of postmenopausal use of estrogen. Additionally, several placebo controlled clinical trials of estrogen therapy for AD have been conducted. As such, we are now in a position to assess the potential for the use of estrogens as a preventative or a disease-modifying treatment of this neurodegenerative disease.

Alzheimer's disease (AD) is a significant personal, family, social, and public health problem. Currently the allopathic medical community maintains that there is no way to prevent or cure AD. The latest opinions on the possibility of hormone replacement therapy (HRT)/ estrogen replacement therapy (ERT) as a means to prevent and treat AD are the most promising and conclusive evidence of the link between the lack of bio-identical hormones and early onset AD that we have seen to date. Although prevention and treatment of AD can now be added to the list of HRT/ERT's benefits, research in the area needs to be widened. The potential benefits include improved interest and compliance with HRT, improved quality of life, and cost savings. The problems include difficulties in monitoring and managing clients with AD, assuring compliance with the therapeutic regimen, and deciding when to withdraw therapy.

Alzheimer's Progestins are a synthetic version of the naturally-occurring female reproductive hormone progesterone. The compounds were initially designed to counteract certain unwanted effects of estrogen in reproductive tissues, particularly in the uterus. Several generations of progestins have been developed both for use in contraception and but bio-identical hormone replacement during menopause seems to be the most promising, as the hidden dangers of synthetic hormone replacement becomes more widely studied.

While the target of progestins used in hormone therapy is generally the uterus, progestin therapy affects every major organ system including the brain, the cardiovascular system, the immune system and the generation of blood cells. As in other systems, progestins have unique effects on the brain which ultimately could impact the long-term neurological health of users. Most of the effects of progestins on the brain are beneficial, although some research has shown that they may pose some risks.

Thyroid dysfunction has been implicated as a cause of reversible cognitive impairment nd as such, the thyroid stimulating hormone has long been part of the screening laboratory test for dementia. Recently, several population-based studies demonstrated an association between hypo- or hyperthyroidism and Alzheimer's disease. This review discusses the role of thyroid hormone in the normal development and regulation of central nervous system functions and summarizes the studies that have linked thyroid function and dementia risk. Finally, it explores possible biological mechanisms to explain this association, including the direct effects of thyroid hormone on cerebral amyloid processing, neurodegeneration and thyrotropin-mediated mechanisms and vascular mediated enhancement of Alzheimer's disease risk.

# TREATMENT RECOMMENDATIONS
## FOR EARLY STAGES OF ALZHEIMER'S DISEASE

———————— ⟨ ⟩ ————————

I BELIEVE IT is possible to recover from the earlier stages of Alzheimer's, if prompt and proper treatment is administered. Unfortunately, when the disease has destroyed too many brain cells, it is too late for patients to recover.

My father was able to recognize family members and was also able to speak in sentences when he began his testosterone, desiccated thyroid, and DHEA.

I believe that the ability to speak in sentences and to recognize family members may prove to be prerequisites for patients to have a chance of recovery, if prompt and proper treatment is administered.

1 – Begin Vitamin D-3. I recommend a blood test (25 hydroxy vitamin D) in order to determine your vitamin D level. Many alternative doctors believe the optimal level should be 65- 70 ng/ml.

2 – Begin Nitric Oxide. *The Nitric Oxide (NO) Solution*, by Nathan Bryan, Ph.D., documents extensive research about how nitric oxide promotes arterial health as well as helping brain cells function more efficiently.

NEOGENIS is the name of the company that that sells NEO-40. Neo-40 raises nitric oxide levels in our bodies by using natural ingredients. I recommend one tablet twice a day for my patients who are suffering from a chronic illness. In my experience, approximately two months of treatment are required to help restore arterial health.

A note of caution: There are several prescription medications that cannot be taken at the same time as NEO-40. These include organic nitrate medications such as nitro-glycerine, isosorbide dinitrate, erectile dysfunction drugs, and blood thinners.

3 — Begin testosterone. Dr. Friedman's research indicates that testosterone supplementation is an excellent third choice to begin for both men and women. Compounding pharmacists can prepare topical creams that contain bio-identical testosterone. Most men will benefit from 50-100 mg (milligrams) daily. Women may begin with 1 to 5 mg of testosterone. If tolerated, some women may benefit from increasing up to 10 mg daily.

A growing number of men and women are opting for bio-identical testosterone implants. The implants are placed under the skin of the buttocks, and gradually release the hormones 24 hours a day.

4 — Dr. Thierry Hertoghe is a world renowned Belgium physician who specializes in endocrinology. He prescribes 200 mg of progesterone nightly for men that suffer from an enlarged prostate (benign prostatic hypertrophy or BPH). After beginning the progesterone, the BPH usually begins to resolve within several weeks. This research indicates that both men and women who suffer from early stages of Alzheimer's may benefit from taking 200 mg of bio-identical progesterone nightly.

5- Dr. Friedman's research showed estradiol is the most potent form of estrogen that will help prevent Alzheimer's disease. The majority of women will benefit from taking one or two mg of estradiol daily.

6 – Begin DHEA. I recommend women begin 10 mg AM and PM. Men require larger dosages. I recommend 25 mg twice daily.

DHEA is a neuroactive steroid that affects the central nervous system (which includes the brain), as well as, the peripheral nervous system. DHEA also impacts the neural circuitry establishing and maintaining new synaptic connections in the brain. Again, this is one of the hormones that helped my father cover.

7 – Cautiously begin bio-identical thyroid hormones. Desiccated thyroid has proven itself to be the most effective form of thyroid for over a century. It was the only form of thyroid utilized in Dr. Barnes' long-term study. I recommend beginning a very small dosage two months after beginning nitric oxide. One-quarter grain every other day is an adequate starting dosage for chronically ill patients. Increase the dosage by the same amount monthly.

Patients who suffer from numerous allergies usually respond better to compounded bio-identical T4 and T3 thyroid hormones.

In my experience, a large number of elderly patients who suffer from chronic illnesses also suffer from numerous allergies. Introducing one hormone at a time will usually reveal an allergic reaction to the hormone. Yes, people may become allergic to their own hormones, especially if they have suffered from chronic mold exposure during their lifetime.

For more details, see the chapter entitled Chronic Mold and Mycotoxins on page X Patients may also have a reaction to the cream or other components that contain the necessary hormones. If this occurs ask your pharmacist to give you samples of a different carrier for the hormones.

Detailed instructions regarding treatment for hypothyroidism are included in the last sections of this book.

**A note of caution:**

**I have treated 100's of elderly patients who have suffered from hypothyroidism and chronic illness. Most of these patients have poor arterial health.**

**Thyroid hormones are among the most powerful medications known to mankind. The heart begins to beat more forcefully after beginning very small dosages of thyroid hormones.**

**If the heart is unable to accommodate the increased blood flow required by the more forceful heartbeats, a heart attack may ensue.**

**Please study and follow the recommendations contained in this book before beginning treatment with thyroid hormones.**

Men and women should seek physicians and clinicians who know how to prescribe bio-identical hormones. I have found that compounding pharmacists are an excellent resource for all those clinicians who want to learn how to prescribe the necessary hormones.

## ADDITIONAL RESEARCH AND INFORMATION

Additional research references that indicate bio-identical hormone therapy helps prevent Alzheimer's disease are included the reference section of this book.

# THE AVAILABILITY OF BIO-IDENTICAL: HORMONES ARE BEING JEOPARDIZED

UNFORTUNATELY, THE PHARMACEUTICAL companies and the FDA have been trying to restrict the ability of compounding pharmacists to dispense bio-identical hormones in America. Pharmaceutical companies are unable obtain patents on our own, natural bio-identical hormones. This restricts them from charging exorbitant fees for these products. As result, they are not interested in producing or promoting bio-identical hormones.

Thankfully, the Congressional Appropriations Committees rejected the FDA's most recent request to restrict compounding pharmacies' ability to dispense bio-identical hormones.

The most resent and most restrictive FDA rules contained even more threats to the ability of practitioners to choose pharmacists who can to prepare individualized and customized therapies.

While completing the last draft of this book in December of 2015, the Congressional Appropriations Committee rejected the FDA's ability to restrict compounding. Their wording reads as follows:

The Congressional Appropriations Committees rejected FDA's request for increased funding to implement the provisions related to compounding within the Drug Quality and Security Act. In addition, the Omnibus appropriations bill expresses grave concern from Congress that FDA has exceeded its authority under the DQSA by prohibiting all office-use compounding and restricting dispensing as well as distribution activities within the Memorandum of Understanding. In order to address these concerns, Congress has included language within the Omnibus appropriations legislation that mandates FDA to release guidance within 90 days of enactment that allows office-use compounding. The Omnibus also contains language that prevents FDA from restricting dispensing of compounded medications within the Memorandum of Understanding and mandates FDA to report to Congress within 90 days as to when the API positive list will be finalized.

This was a great victory for the compounding pharmacies and the consumers who use them. It was the collective efforts of their trade associations, pharmacists, and lobbying efforts that made this possible.

The ever-increasing success of bio-identical hormone therapies illustrates that consumers no longer buy into "the magic bullet" or "one drug treats all" practice of medicine. Indeed, why use a drug instead of addressing a hormone deficiency? Consumers must take every opportunity to insist upon preserving the right to choose personalized solutions.

Our populace needs to keep the government out of our personal relationships with health care providers. Contact your legislators to demand that we retain our ability to be treated using natural, bio-identical hormones.

# BIO-IDENTICAL HORMONES ARE PROVEN TO BE SAFE

D R. F RIEDMAN'S BOOK contains the most comprehensive explanation about why doctors mistakenly believe that giving hormones to women places them at a higher risk to develop cancer.

A major study was begun in 1991 to determine how female hormone replacement medications affected women's general health and longevity. This study was named the Women's Health Initiative (WHI). Dr. Friedman explains why this study was an enormous setback to medical science.

Briefly, the hormones that were given to the participants in the study were not bio-identical. Bio-identical hormones are the exact duplicate of our own hormones, which have been available through compounding pharmacies for decades.

Horse estrogens and synthetic progestins (an artificial form of progesterone) were used in the WHI study. The horse estrogens and synthetic progestins are what almost all conventional doctors have been prescribing for many decades.

Prior to this research study, scientists and doctors assumed that horse estrogens and synthetic progestins worked the same as human estrogen and progesterone within our bodies. Unfortunately, the women in the

WHI study who were prescribed these foreign hormones were found to have a higher risk of developing various cancers, as compared to the group of women who had not taken these hormones. The women who had taken these hormones also had an increased risk of developing a stroke. The control group of women had been given placebos. Placebos looked identical to the drugs that were used, but the pills did not contain any medicine.

This flawed study resulted in millions of women discontinuing their hormone therapies, including those taking bio-identical hormones. Doctors around the world were erroneously taught that all hormones for women increased the risk of breast cancer and strokes.

Bio-identical hormone therapies have now proven themselves to be safe. In 2008, the E3N Cohort Study followed 80,377 for 8.1 years. It verified that medroxyprogesterone (MPA), which is not a bio-identical hormone, was dangerous and resulted in a 48% increase in the rate of invasive breast cancer, compared to the control group, who did not receive the MPA. The women who were given bio-identical hormone therapy had no increase in the rate of invasive breast cancer.

Again, I must emphasize that our own hormones, when utilized properly, are among the most beneficial treatments known to mankind.

My teacher, Dr. Sonkin, related the story of one of his patients who was suffering menopausal symptoms. After alleviating her menopausal symptoms, she asked Dr. Sonkin what she should do with her life. She had divorced her husband and her children had become estranged.

# ELEVATED CHOLESTEROL: INDICATES HYPOTHYROIDISM

DR. BARNES CHECKED cholesterol levels on all of his study patients. Ninety-five percent of the patients who had elevated cholesterol upon entering his study had their cholesterol levels normalize, following proper treatment for their hypothyroidism. He stated that the five percent of patients who continued to have elevated cholesterol did not have an increased risk of having a heart attack.

For the first half of the 20<sup>th</sup> century, doctors were aware that elevated cholesterol was virtually diagnostic of hypothyroidism. In 1934, Dr. L.M. Hurxthal from the Lahey Clinic found the relation of cholesterol to the basal metabolic rate (BMR) was so sensitive, he suggested using serum cholesterol as the diagnostic test for hypothyroidism. e BMR was the first test doctors used to diagnose hypothyroidism.

Thyroid hormones control the rate of our metabolism and our metabolic rate.

My cholesterol and triglyceride levels were well within normal ranges at age 36, during my third year of medical school. Medical students practiced drawing each others' blood, while learning important lessons about blood tests. I believed my scores were normal because I exercised regularly and ate a healthful diet.

By age 41, without any change in diet or exercise, my cholesterol level had risen to 300 and my triglycerides were over 400. My symptoms of hypothyroidism had markedly worsened. Fortunately, Dr. Sonkin placed me on thyroid hormones. Shortly thereafter, my symptoms began to resolve. My elevated cholesterol and triglycerides normalized after 18 months of proper thyroid treatment.

# THE IMPORTANCE OF CHOLESTEROL

It is my opinion that Dr. Jerry Tennant is one of the most gifted physicians on our planet. I believe the most comprehensive research regarding cholesterol and the failure of statin drugs to reduce heart attacks is found in his book, *Healing is Voltage: The Handbook - 3rd Edition*

I recommend his book to everyone. His research is causing a paradigm shift among a rapidly growing number of progressive doctors and scientists.

Dr. Tennant teaches us that all chronic disease is due to the bodies' inability to make healthy new cells. Our bodies are governed by voltage. We must generate enough voltage in order to make healthy new cells. Proper treatment for those with low thyroid function will require additional thyroid hormones in order to supply this vital energy.

Our cells are constantly wearing out and need to be replaced.

We replace every cell in our skin every six weeks, every cell in our liver every eight weeks, and the lining of our gut every two or three days.

Our brain is about 60% fat. Every nerve cell in our brain contains about 50% cholesterol. We must have an ample supply of cholesterol in order to make healthy new cells.

I have included information from the Weston A. Price Foundation that offers crucial research with regard to the importance of healthy cholesterol in our diet. *(See Appendix D in order to read this vital information. Weston A. Price).*

# THE ROLE OF EFA'S

IT IS GENERALLY accepted that lifestyle and particularly dietary habits influence mental health, and prevalence and progression of AD. Numerous epidemiological studies have revealed profitable effects of dietary intake of especially fish oil on cognitive decline during aging and dementia.

Another result of the low-fat dietary belief was the replacement of fats in the diet with refined carbohydrates, which leads to a rise in blood glucose levels and over time to insulin resistance and diabetes. They point out that the prevalence of fructose, mostly in the form of high fructose corn syrup, is ten times more reactive than glucose in inducing glycation (for a detailed discussion of this, see the video below: "5 Medical Doctors with Gary Taubes and Robb Wolf Discuss Coconut Oil and Alzheimer's Disease".) This impairs serum proteins, and they hypothesize that this leads to a depletion of much needed cholesterol and fat in the brain. Strong evidence in favor of their hypothesis is the fact that studies show patients with type-2 diabetes are at two to five times increased risk to AD.

Increased lipid peroxidation is also shown to be an early cause of Alzheimer's disease. Liquid vegetable oils, the polyunsaturates, are highly prone to oxidation and rancidity, and it is now well known that in the form of trans fatty acids (through the process of hydrogenation) they are extremely toxic.

*Coconut oil, by contrast, is highly saturated, and in its natural unrefined form has a shelf life of more than 2 years. Unlike unsaturated oils, it is not prone to oxidation.*

As coconut oil's use becomes more accepted and widespread, and as people begin to realize the dangers of the low-fat dietary belief, we are starting to see more testimonies in relation to diseases like Alzheimer's. One of the most widely published reports is from Dr. Mary Newport as reported by the St. Petersburg Times on October 29, 2008[6]. Dr. Newport's husband had been diagnosed with early onset Alzheimer's and was watching her husband quickly deteriorate. After using drugs that slowed down the effects of Alzheimer's, she looked into clinical drug trials and found one based on MCTs that not only slowed the progression of Alzheimer's, but offered *improvement*. Not being able to get her husband into one of these trials, she began to give him Virgin Coconut Oil, and saw incredible improvement in his condition.

The coconut oil he'd ingested seemed to "lift the fog." He began taking coconut oil every day, and by the fifth day, there was a tremendous improvement. "He would face the day bubbly, more like his old self," his wife said. More than five months later, his tremors subsided, the visual disturbances that prevented him from reading disappeared, and he became more social and interested in those around him.

# CONCLUSION:
## ALZHEIMER'S DISEASE CAN BE PREVENTED

DR.BRODA BARNES AND I have had profound success preventing Alzheimer's disease in our patients for more than thirty years. My father's recovery from mild to moderate Alzheimer's disease at age 82 bodes well for all those who have begun to display symptoms that are associated with the illness. I hope and pray that our doctors and compounding pharmacists will be allowed to utilize the information presented in this book.

# THE WESTON A PRICE FOUNDATION HEALTHFUL FAT DIET

THE WESTON A Price Foundation provides a wealth of information regarding the vital importance "good fats" in our diet.

According to research from the Weston A. Price Foundation, humans need saturated fats such as cholesterol to have optimal healthy bodies. Studies have shown that there is no correlation between cholesterol levels in our blood and heart disease.

Scientific studies on fat in clogged arteries revealed that only 26% is saturated fat and the rest is unsaturated fats. Cholesterol does not cause disease. More importantly, it plays an important role in the body chemistry as summarized in the following statements: Saturated fats include cholesterol, which constitute 50% of the cell membranes that provide the necessary stiffness and integrity that our cells need to properly function.

Saturated fats lower lipoprotein A (Lp(A) which is used as a marker for heart disease.

They protect the liver from alcohol and medications such as Tylenol.

Higher levels of cholesterol enhance our immune system and protect us against infections of all kinds.

Essential fatty acids (EFAs) such as Omega-3 are better retained in the tissues when there are higher levels of saturated fats in our diet.

The heart stores saturated fat such as 16-carbon palmitic acid to use in times of stress.

Short and medium-chain saturated fatty acids are antimicrobial and protect our digestive tract from harmful microorganisms.

Dietary cholesterol is important for the health of our gut. Studies have shown low cholesterol and vegetarian diets may cause leaky gut syndrome and other intestinal disorders.

Cholesterol is important in the production of corticosteroids and sex hormones like testosterone, estrogen and progesterone. These hormones help us deal with stress and protect us from heart disease and cancer.

Cholesterol is a precursor to vitamin D, a very important fat-soluble vitamin needed for healthy bones and a healthy nervous system. Vitamin D also promotes proper growth, mineral metabolism, proper muscle tone, insulin production, normal reproduction, and immune system function.

Recent research shows that cholesterol behaves as an antioxidant, protecting us against free radical damage, which is a leading cause of heart disease and cancer.

Serotonin receptors found in the brain require cholesterol to function properly. Low cholesterol levels have been linked to increased aggressive and violent behavior, as well as depression and suicidal tendencies.

Babies require high levels of cholesterol for proper brain and nervous system development.

Our brains need saturated fats and cholesterol for memory. In fact, seniors with the highest cholesterol levels have the best memory function.

Individuals with hypothyroidism will often have high cholesterol levels. When thyroid function is poor, usually from a diet high in sugar and low in iodine and fat-soluble vitamins and other nutrients, the body floods the blood with cholesterol as a protective mechanism and providing the cells with materials needed for tissue repair and production of protective steroids. Hypothyroid individuals are at a high risk for developing infections, heart disease and cancer.

In summary saturated fats such as butter, meat fats, coconut oil and palm oil are needed in our diets for optimal health and function and are not the blame for our modern diseases such as heart disease, cancer, obesity, diabetes and nervous disorders. It is the advent of modern processed vegetable oil that is associated with the epidemic of modern degenerative disease not the consumption of saturated fats.

# VITAMIN B12

ONE OF THE more common problems that I have seen in my patient population is that dementia may be due to a vitamin B12 deficiency. Proper treatment using Vitamin B 12 helps ensure that this deficiency does not cause serious cognitive problems, and helps avoid a host of other chronic illnesses.

There are two books on the subject that I highly recommend. The first book is entitled: *Could It Be B12: An Epidemic of Misdiagnosis.* The second book is: *Vitamin B12 for Your Health.*

Both books document that the blood tests doctors use to evaluate patients' Vitamin B12 status are not accurate. The blood tests are erroneous and do not reflect whether or not patients require supplementation with vitamin B12.

A large percentage of the population is unable to assimilate B12 orally. Many of these people need to take B12 under their tongue *(sublingually).* More severely affected people need to have regular injections. Dementia caused by B12 deficiency is usually treatable.

The following is a compilation of the research in these two books as well as what I have learned over the years.

# B12 DEFICIENCY SYMPTOMS INCLUDE:

Depression
Mania
Paranoia
Irritability
Delusions
Schizophrenic symptoms
Personality changes
Anemia
Brain fog
Bursitis
Depression
Fatigue
Fibromyalgia
Heart disease
Dementia

# RISK OF B12 DEFICIENCY:

Vegetarians

60+ years old

Hypothyroidism

Had gastric or intestinal surgery

Antacids, metfomin, and related diabetes drugs that block absorption

Anorexia, bulimia

Alcoholism

Celiac disease, Crohn's disease, IBS (irritable bowel syndrome)

Autoimmune, Hashimoto's, Graves' disease

Dental procedures that use nitrous oxide

> Nitrous oxide (laughing gas) is often used in dental procedures to sedate patients. The nitrous oxide depletes almost all of the patients' B12. I have seen elderly dental patients who were profoundly affected and their dentist was unaware of the cause.

# DRUG-INDUCED B12 DEFICIENCY

H2 blockers (all of which reduce stomach acid) and antacids are worst offenders
Colchicine
Biguanides - Metformin
Phenytoin
Potassium chloride (K-Dur)
Para-aminosalicylates (Paser, anti-TB)
Cholestyramine

Dr. Brownstein's current recommendations are to begin a trial of vitamin B12 injections for everyone who suffers from the previously listed symptoms.

Dr. Brownstein recommends that patients should begin an injection of 1 milligram daily for 30 days. Subcutaneous (under the skin) or intramuscular (IM) injections are equally affective. The form of vitamin B12 that he recommends is called hydroxycobalamin.

After treating 1,000s of patients, hydoxocobalamin has shown to be the most beneficial form.

I recommend a different form of B12 injections for my patients that suffer from severe allergies. It is called methylcobalamin. Compounding pharmacies can provide preservative free methylcobalamin. It is injected under the skin (subcutaneous) or into the muscle (intramuscular). If the patients' symptoms do not improve within 30 days, the vitamin B12 trial is discontinued.

Dr. Brownstein stated that 80% of his patients' who follow his protocol will realize significant improvement in their health.

For those who realize improvement, he recommends a maintenance dosage of 1 mg injected twice a week. Dr. Brownstein has reversed a number of patients who were suffering early forms of dementia.

Vitamin B12 is water soluble, which means it is easily eliminated from the body and rarely causes any side effects. Occasionally, patients who suffer from numerous allergies may develop an allergic reaction to the injection site. Patients with more severe allergies may not tolerate this treatment.

# CHRONIC MOLD AND MYCOTOXINS

MOLD AND MYCOTOXINS usually interfere with proper thyroid treatment and are the root cause of numerous other allergies.

The majority of my patients who suffer from mold allergies and mold toxins are unable to tolerate a therapeutic dosage of thyroid. Many of these patients feel better when taking a very small dosage of thyroid. However, when the dosage of thyroid hormones is gradually increased, these patients develop palpitations, tremors, and feel worse instead of better.

Younger, healthier patients may tolerate a therapeutic dosage of thyroid. However, if they continue to be exposed to mold, they may have to decrease or stop the thyroid because they become jittery or develop palpitations.

Dr.William J. Rea is the number one environmental medicine doctor in the world. His clinic is in Dallas Texas (ehcd.com). He taught me that patients who suffer from mold toxins may become allergic to their own hormones. I see such patients frequently. These toxins also cause numerous other allergies and decrease patients' immunity. Such patients are often unaware of the fact that they have developed numerous food sensitivities and other environmental allergies. Recurrent infections frequently occur.

It is my opinion that a treatment called "provocative neutralization" offers patients the best chance to resolve mold and hormone allergies.

Mold and hormone allergy testing is performed by injecting a tiny amount of each type of mold under the skin. Five minutes are allowed to pass in order to document the symptoms and severity of the reaction for each type of mold. The mold testing takes approximately two days before the proper treatment may be administered.

There are dozens of different types of mold. I had reactions to all of the molds that were tested, which meant that I had developed allergies to all of the molds.

Treatment involves making a homeopathic dilution for each type of mold to which the patient had a reaction. This dilution neutralizes the mold toxins, which allows the body to heal. Patients take a very small injection of the homeopathic dilution every four days.

Homeopathy has proven itself to be a wonderful alternative treatment modality for hundreds of years.

Most patients require six months to one year of treatment in order for their mold allergies to resolve. Mold immunotherapy involves injecting a very small amount under the skin every four days. Additionally, people who suffer from severe mold allergies must find a mold free home or workplace, if they expect to fully recover. Those who are unable to remove themselves from the moldy environment may be relieved from fifty percent of their symptoms but are not likely to completely recover.

There are several other environmental allergy clinics in America that offer provocative neutralization. There is also one such clinic in Great Britain.

You may contact Dr. Rea's clinic for more information. Unfortunately, his clinic does not accept insurance. His methods are not considered to be" *The Standard of Care."* Which is defined as:

1. *Diagnostic and treatment process that a clinician should follow for a certain type of patient, illness, or clinical circumstance. Adjuvant chemotherapy for lung cancer is "a new standard of care, but not necessarily the only standard of care". (New England Journal of Medicine, 2004)*
2. *In legal terms, the level at which an ordinary, prudent professional with the same training and experience in good standing in a same or similar community would practice under the same or similar circumstances. An "average" standard would not apply because in that case at least half of any group of practitioners would not qualify. The medical malpractice plaintiff must establish the appropriate standard of care and demonstrate that the standard of care has been breached, with expert testimony.*

It is because of these restrictions that I moved to Arizona, in order to obtain my MD(H) medical license. My homeopathic medical board has a different view of what should be considered *the standard of care*. As long as I can produce proven research that has been previously documented in medical journals and text books, and my patient's outcomes are far superior to the allopathic model, my medical board supports my method of practicing medicine

The American Environmental Health Foundation (aehf.com) offers the best method to test for mold spores in the home or place of work. If mold spores are found growing in your home, you have a problem. Collecting mold spores out of the air is a very poor second choice. Everyone must take precautions when removing mold. I told one of my patients that I believed she had a mold problem in her home. She found black mold, which is the most toxic of all the molds, and removed it without taking any precautions. She suffered acute kidney failure following her removal of the black mold. Mold removal must be done by professionals.

# RECOMMENDED READING LIST

Barnes BO. *Hypothyroidism, The Unsuspected Illness.* Harper. 1976.

Brownstein D. *The Statin Disaster.* Medical Alternatives Press. Available at: www.drbrownstein.com/The-Statin-Disaster-p/statindisaster.htm

Brownstein D. *Vitamin B12 for Your Health.* Medical Alternatives Press. 2012.

Colborn T, Dumanoski D. *Our Stolen Future: Are We Threatening Our Fertility, Intelligence, and Survival?—A Scientific Detective Story.* Plume. 1997.

Freidman E, Cain W. *The New Testosterone Treatment: How You and Your Doctor Can Fight Breast Cancer, Prostate Cancer, and Alzheimer's.* Prometheus Books. 2013.

Pacholok SM, Stuart JJ. *Could It Be B12: An Epidemic of Misdiagnosis.* Quill Driver Books; 2nd ed. edition. 2011.

Solomon M. *Living Well with Graves' Disease and Hyperthyroidism: What Your Doctor Doesn't Tell You...That You Need to Know.* William Morrow Paperbacks. 2005.

Starr M. *How to Prevent Heart Attacks, Heart Failure, Diabetes.* New Voice Publications. 2013.

Starr M. *Hypothyroidism Type 2: The Epidemic — Revised Edition.* New Voice Publications. 2013.

Tennant J. *Healing is Voltage: The Handbook - 3rd Edition.* CreateSpace Independent Publishing Platform. 2010.

# DIAGNOSIS AND PROPER TREATMENT FOR HYPOTHYROIDISM

———— ⟨◝◞⟩ ————

THE FOLLOWING INFORMATION is contained in my second book *Heart Attacks, Heart Failure, and Diabetes.* I have repeated much of this information in order to provide comprehensive thyroid research and treatment.

## WHY THE TSH BLOOD TEST IS INACCURATE AND SHOULD BE ABANDONED

The TSH blood test was invented in the 1960s and became the "standard of care" in 1971. Currently, the normal blood test values range from 0.4 to 4.6 in America. These values have changed several times and differ in other countries. If the TSH is above 4.6, the patient is diagnosed to be hypothyroid.

If the TSH test is in the normal range, no matter how many hypothyroid symptoms people suffer, doctors are taught that their symptoms could not possibly result from hypothyroidism.

Doctors are taught that the TSH is elevated when our bodies need more thyroid hormones. If the TSH result is below normal (suppressed), doctors are taught that the patient is taking an overdose of thyroid hormones. Another reason why the TSH may be suppressed is because the patient may have hyperthyroidism, which is also called Graves' disease. Graves' disease occurs if the thyroid gland is producing too many thyroid hormones.

The following description and illustration should help to clarify how TSH is produced.

There are several physiological assumptions on which the validity of blood tests for hypothyroidism depends (see corresponding numbers in the following diagram):

1.  The peripheral tissues transmit their need for thyroid hormones to the brain.
2.  The part of the brain called the hypothalamus transmits these signals to another part of the brain called the pituitary gland.
3.  The pituitary secretes TSH (thyroid stimulating hormone), which gives the signal to the thyroid gland to secrete more thyroid hormones.
4.  The thyroid gland secretes thyroid hormones.
5.  Thyroid hormones are transported to the peripheral tissues via the blood.

Doctors have been taught that the action of the thyroid hormones on the tissues reduces the demand for more thyroid hormones. However, research was published in 2012 that indicated that the pituitary gland has a unique enzyme that works independently from the rest of the body.

Research Indicates Why the TSH Test Should No Longer Be Used for Testing and Treating Hypothyroidism

A research study was published in January 2012 by the National Academy of Hypothyroidism an alternative group of thyroid specialists) that provided strong evidence that the TSH blood test is not an accurate measurement of our body's thyroid function. REF 15 in HA book

Figure 1

**Thyroid Pathways**

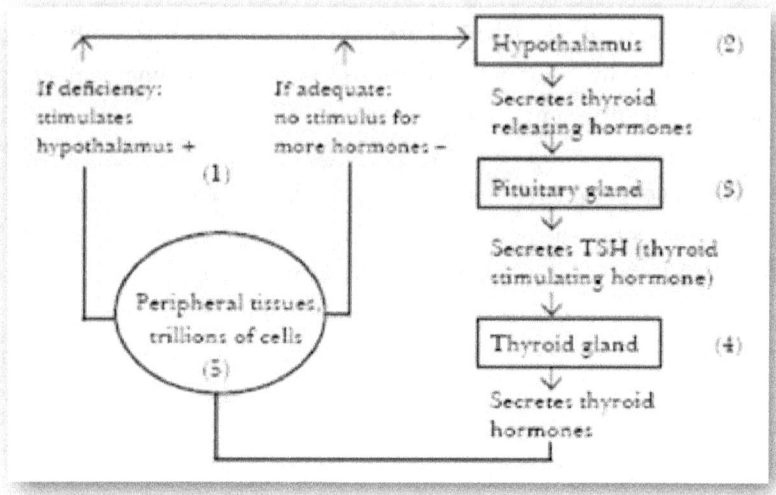

In order to simplify this research data, I must first explain how the body utilizes thyroid hormones. There are four different forms of our own thyroid hormones. They are named T4, T3, T2, and T1. The predominant form of thyroid secreted from our thyroid gland contains four iodine molecules and is called T4. The "T" is an amino acid named tyrosine, which is in all four forms of our thyroid. T4 is a relatively weak hormone and must be converted into T3 by an enzyme named deiodinase (de means to remove). This enzyme removes one iodine molecule and converts T4 into T3. T3 has about five times more physiological activity than T4. T2 is necessary for acute increased needs for energy. T1 has much less activity.

This new research revealed that there are three different forms of deiodinases that are named D-1, D-2, and D-3. These enzymes function semi-independently. D-1 converts T4 into T3 throughout the body but is not a significant determinant of the conversion of T4 to T3 in the pituitary. The TSH is produced in the pituitary.

D-1 is suppressed and down regulated in response to physiological and emotional stress, depression, dieting, weight gain, insulin resistance, obesity, diabetes, leptin resistance, autoimmune diseases, systemic illness, chronic fatigue, fibromyalgia, chronic pain, and exposure to toxins and plastics. In such conditions, there are reduced tissue levels of T3 everywhere in the body except the pituitary gland (which was previously unknown).

The reduced tissue levels of T3 throughout the body have previously been quoted as a beneficial response that lowers tissue metabolism. There is no evidence to justify this claim. However, there is significant evidence demonstrating a detrimental response to the lower T3 levels.

D-2 is produced by the pituitary and is regulated by intra-pituitary T3 levels. Pituitary T3 levels usually do not correlate or provide an accurate indicator of T3 levels in the rest of the body.

The pituitary is different from every other tissue in the body. There is a unique make up of deiodinases in the pituitary that often respond opposite to that of other tissues in the body.

Numerous conditions result in an increase in pituitary T3 while simultaneously suppressing T3 in the rest of the body. Again, these conditions are physiological and emotional stress, depression, dieting, weight gain, insulin resistance, obesity, diabetes, leptin resistance, autoimmune diseases, systemic illness, chronic fatigue, fibromyalgia, chronic pain, and exposure to toxins and plastics.

Pituitary T3 levels are determined by D-2 activity, which is 1,000 times more efficient at converting T4 to T3 than the D-1 enzyme in the rest of the body and is much less sensitive to suppression by toxins and medications. In the pituitary, 80-90% of T4 is converted to T3 while only about 30-50% of T4 in the peripheral tissue is converted into active T3.

The pituitary levels of T3 are under completely different physiological control than the rest of the body. Pituitary levels of T3 will always be significantly higher than anywhere else in the body.

This research clearly shows that the TSH blood test should not be used to diagnose and treat hypothyroidism. Unfortunately, this research has not been published in mainstream endocrinology journals or textbooks.

# BASAL METABOLIC RATE

*In order to help you understand Dr. Sonkin's research, I will explain a test named Basal Metabolic Rate (BMR).*

Thyroid hormones control the speed and efficiency of our metabolism. Hypothyroidism slows down our metabolism. The BMR test was developed in the early 20th century to help aid doctors with the often difficult and obscure diagnosis of hypothyroidism.

The test measured a person's metabolism by monitoring oxygen consumption for a given height, weight, age, and sex. Normal values were determined from a large number of apparently healthy people. However, in order for the BMR to be accurate, the patient must be free from stress and nervous tension. Tension can result from chronic pain, neuroses, anxiety, or other problems associated with hypothyroidism.

Patients were tested after a good night sleep. They were instructed to fast after their evening meal and to travel immediately to the test location upon awakening. If they lived too far away, they were hospitalized overnight in an attempt to ensure accuracy. A tight clip was placed on their nose and a tube inserted into their mouth to measure oxygen. Stressors and tension often resulted in a normal or above average BMR despite the fact that a patient's metabolism was actually low. A British study tested 100 patients with definite hypothyroidism in 1960. The BMR test confirmed the illness in only 77 of the patients.

In 1998, I recruited a Ph.D. exercise physiologist to perform basal metabolic rate testing for my pain patients. The doctor was very conscientious and tried to make certain the patients were relaxed and proper procedures followed. He performed basal metabolism tests on 50 consecutive pain patients. All of these patients had normal TSH blood tests.

My 50 patients' metabolism averaged 15% below normal. A significant number of their metabolic rates were in the 30–40% below normal range. Several tests were above average as well. When a basal metabolism test was previously used to aid doctors in making the diagnosis of hypothyroidism, a test result of 10% less than normal or lower was considered strongly indicative of the illness.

I sent copies of the low basal metabolic tests to the patients' primary care physicians along with my diagnosis of hypothyroidism. Almost without exception, the test results as well as the patients' textbook symptomatology were ignored. Their physicians simply felt that the TSH blood tests could not be wrong.

An unfortunate 80 year-old woman held the record low metabolism for all my patients. She initially was unable to stay awake during her office visits and summoned all her energy to travel to and from my office. The patient stated she slept for most of the previous 10 years after a new doctor stopped her thyroid medication. The doctor said her blood tests showed that she no longer needed thyroid hormones. Despite the fact she had taken the hormones for over 40 years, and was doing quite well, the thyroid hormones were stopped. Her BMR showed that her metabolic rate was 48% below normal, even though her TSH was in the normal range.

The test results from my patients and Dr. Sonkin's patients indicate that the TSH does not measure patients' metabolic rate (BMR). There are no studies in any of the medical literature showing that such a correlation exists.

Dr. Sonkin's research also illustrates how normal thyroid blood tests do not measure the BMR and are missing untold numbers of patients suffering from hypothyroidism.

Figure 2

Therapeutic Trials (TSH and/or T-4 normal)

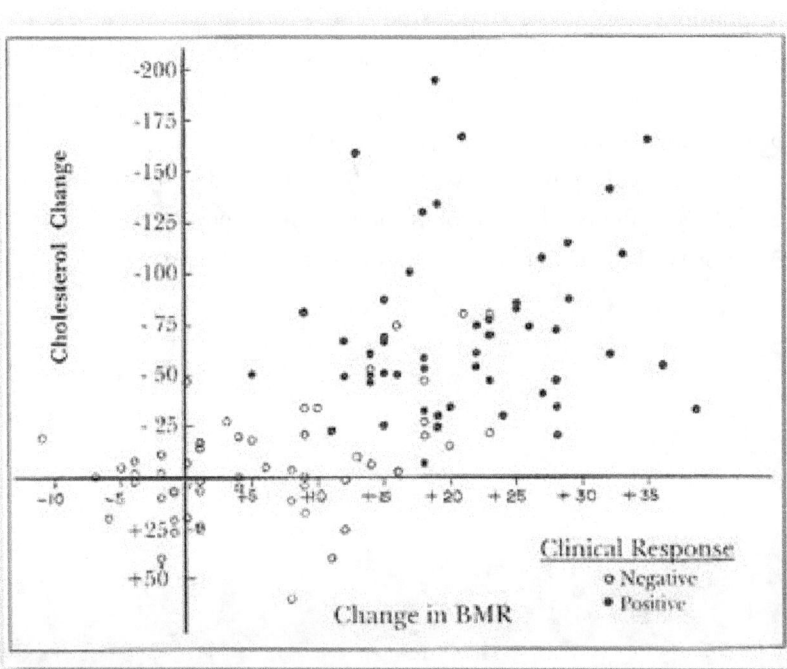

Source: Gelb H. *Clinical Management of Head, Neck, and TMJ\* Pain and Dysfunction.* Philadelphia: W. B. Saunders, 1977; page 162. Reprinted with permission.

- Temporomandibular joint (TMJ) pain is another symptom of hypothyroidism.

The graph illustrates how many of Dr. Sonkin's patients with normal thyroid blood tests responded well to thyroid hormones. One hundred consecutive patients with symptoms of hypothyroidism were tested. The change in BMR and cholesterol levels was plotted on the graph. The patients represented by the darkened circles reported improvement of their symptoms. The patients represented by the clear circles reported no improvement in their symptoms (negative clinical response).

The horizontal line represents the change in BMR after a trial of thyroid hormones (a combination of T3 and T4). Two-thirds (66/100) of the patients' BMRs increased from 10% to 35%. The vertical line represents the drop in patients' cholesterol. Following treatment, over half of the patients' cholesterol dropped from 25 points to 200 points. A majority of the patients' hypothyroid symptoms improved.

# 24 HOUR URINE T3 TEST

Dr. Jacques Hertoghe, the 3rd generation endocrinologist, developed an accurate test to detect hypothyroidism. It is called the 24-hour urine T3 test and measures how much of the active form of thyroid (T3) is excreted in 24 hours. The Hertoghe method of testing and treatment is desperately needed around the world.

Dr. Jacques Hertoghe and two of his colleagues did the following study. Two groups of patients were treated for hypothyroidism. The first group of patients had already been diagnosed with hypothyroidism and placed on T4 by other doctors. They sought help at the clinic because the T4 treatments did not relieve their symptoms. The second group of patients had never been treated for hypothyroidism. They went to the Hertoghe clinic because they were ailing and hoped to get help for their ailments. These doctors and the senior Hertoghes had been using desiccated thyroid and treating hypothyroidism quite successfully for most of the 20th century.

In the 1970s, doctors in all the western nations were instructed to begin treating thyroid blood tests with the new synthetic T4 instead of treating patients with desiccated thyroid (that had worked quite well since the late 19th century). It did not take long for Dr. Hertoghe and his colleagues to realize that this new method of treatment was a very poor substitute for their former method, which emphasized resolution of patients' symptoms using desiccated thyroid. They stated, "It is necessary to stress that the clinical evaluation of the patient's condition must precede interpretation of laboratory tests and not follow it." Figure 3 highlights eight of the most common symptoms of hypothyroidism. Symptoms were measured before and after their treatment. These doctors wanted to show how well the patients' symptoms responded using treatments they had used for decades, versus the relatively new mandated treatment with synthetic thyroid.

Figure 3 Score of Symptoms under T4 and under
NDT (Natural Desiccated Thyroid)

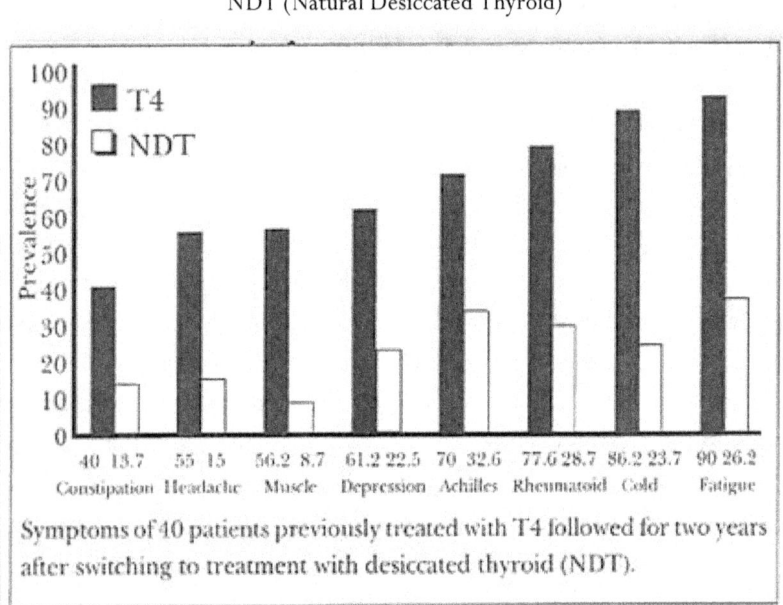

Symptoms of 40 patients previously treated with T4 followed for two years after switching to treatment with desiccated thyroid (NDT).

Source: Hertoghe J, Baiser WV, Eeckhaut W. Thyroid insufficiency. Is thyroxine the only valuable drug? *J Nutr Environ Med.* 2001; 11:159-166. Reprinted with permission.

The patients represented by the dark bar graph had previously been treated for hypothyroidism by other doctors. These other doctors had prescribed synthetic T4, which is one the most commonly prescribed medications in the world. Brand names of T4 include Synthroid®, Levoxyl®, levothyroxine, and Unithroid®.

Patients in the Hertoghe study who had been taking T4 were not relieved of their symptoms and sought help from the Belgian clinic. The 89 patients who had been taking T4 were switched to desiccated thyroid. Symptoms from 40 of the 89 patients were followed for about two years. The patients' symptoms markedly improved after treatment with natural desiccated thyroid (NDT).

The white bar graph represents the patients' symptoms following treatment with natural desiccated thyroid. Fatigue decreased from 90% to 26%. Cold intolerance decreased from 86% to 23%. Rheumatoid means joint and muscle pain, and was decreased from 77% to 28%. Achilles is a reflex at the back of the ankle that is often sluggish when hypothyroidism is present. Sluggish reflexes reduced from 70% to 32%. Depression decreased from 61% to 22%. Muscle cramps decreased from 56% to 8%. Headaches and migraines decreased from 55% to 15%. Constipation decreased from 40% to 13% in this group of patients.

The second page of this study includes 278 patients who had not been previously treated (see Table 1). They were also given desiccated thyroid and followed for about two years. They responded equally well.

The dosages of desiccated thyroid that were given to patients in this study ranged from 2 grains of desiccated thyroid to 5 grains. These dosages are exactly the same as the ones in Dr. Barnes' long-term study to prevent heart attacks. The average adult dosage for the T4 treated patients was 233 mg (or about 3.5 grains) and the untreated group required an average of 200 mg (about 3 grains) for most of their symptoms to resolve. Patients were followed for about two years because thyroid hormones continue to improve patients' symptoms over that length of time.

Table 1

Symptoms Score of T4 Treated Patients Who Were Subsequently Treated with Natural Desiccated Thyroid (NDT)

| | Untreated | | T4 Treated | |
| | 832 | 278 | 89 | 40 |
|---|---|---|---|---|
| Symptoms score | 10.0 | 10.1 | 10.4 | 10.7 |
| Urine T3 pmol | 756.0 | 752.0 | 767.0 | 797.5 |
| Months of treatment | | | 38.6 | 33.2 |
| Thyroxine ug | | | 97.6 | 99.7 |
| | | NDT treated 278 | | NDT treated 40 |
| Symptoms score | | 3.6 | | 3.6 |
| Urine T3 pmol | | 1900.0 | | 1900.0 |
| Months of ug treatment | | 23.0 | | 26.9 |
| NDT mg | | 200.0 | | 233.0 |

The maximum possible score for symptoms was 16. Pmol (picomol) and ug (microgram) are units of measure. NDT is natural desiccated thyroid.

The maximum possible score for symptoms was 16.
Pmol (picomol) and mcg (microgram) are units of measure.
NDT is natural desiccated thyroid.

Source: Hertoghe J, Baiser WV, Eeckhaut W. Thyroid insufficiency.
Is thyroxine the only valuable drug? *J Nutr Environ Med.* 2001;
11:159-166. Reprinted with permission.

Another doctor had previously diagnosed patients in the T4 treated group with hypothyroidism because their TSH was elevated. When the TSH is elevated, the thyroid gland is producing very few thyroid hormones. These patients usually require a slightly higher dosage of thyroid versus the untreated group. Other doctors had not previously diagnosed the untreated group because they had normal TSH blood tests. The untreated group required 200 mg NDT versus 233 mg in the T4 treated group.

Dr. Hertoghe and his colleagues knew that the TSH blood test was erroneous and successfully treated these patients based on their symptoms and the 24-hour urine test.

*I tell my patients that thyroid treatment is measured in months and years, not days and weeks.*

My clinical experience using desiccated thyroid is quite similar to the findings in this study. These dosages are exactly what I have prescribed to restore my patients' health. The average adult dosage is 3 to 3.5 grains per day. The larger the person, the more thyroid they require to regain their health. There are always exceptions, especially if the patient's thyroid gland has been removed or destroyed by radioactive iodine, or other medications. These patients require much larger dosages.

# MY CLINICAL EXPERIENCE

I BEGAN MY pain clinic in 1996, and within two years I realized the vast majority of my pain patients suffered from hypothyroidism. I decided to review my pain patients' medical histories, symptoms, and physical findings after realizing the pervasiveness of hypothyroidism in my pain patients. Random chart reviews were preformed on 162 adult patients out of over 500 patients. Table 2 lists my patients' symptoms associated with hypothyroidism. There were 44 males and 118 females. Their average age was 49 years.

In Table 3, I separated 34 patients who were already being treated for hypothyroidism (with T4) out of the 162 patients.

Starr Pain Clinic Patients: 162 Chart Reviews

| | Number of Patients | Percentage |
|---|---|---|
| Pain | 156 | 96 |
| Dry Skin | 157 | 83 |
| Fatigue | 134 | 83 |
| Brittle/Ridged Nails | 131 | 81 |
| Menstrual problems (females) | 81 | 69 |
| Depression | 91 | 57 |
| Myxedema: | | |
| Moderate to Marked | 88 | 54 |
| Cold Intolerance | 86 | 53 |
| Insomnia | 86 | 53 |
| Delayed Ankle Reflexes | 80 | 49 |
| Hysterectomy (females) | 43 | 41 |
| Allergies | 66 | 41 |
| Cold Hands or Feet | 62 | 38 |
| Weight Gain | 61 | 38 |
| Constipation | 52 | 32 |
| High Blood Pressure | 50 | 31 |
| Tension (anxiety) | 47 | 29 |
| Headaches | 46 | 28 |
| Hair Loss | 45 | 28 |
| TMJ-Teeth Clenching | 40 | 25 |
| Paresthesias (tingling) | 58 | 24 |
| Hypothyroidism, Type 1 | 34 | 21 |
| Tremor | 31 | 19 |
| Heart Disease | 27 | 17 |
| Diabetes | 26 | 16 |
| Heat Intolerance | 25 | 15 |
| Cancer | 15 | 9 |
| Autoimmune Disease | 12 | 7 |
| Hypoglycemia | 11 | 7 |
| Emphysema | 8 | 5 |

Starr Pain Clinic Patients with Prior Diagnosis of Hypothyroidism

*Already Receiving Treatment (T4, i.e., levothyroxine), dosage range 0.1 mg (100 mcg) to 0.2 mg (200 mcg) per day.*

Patients in Table 3, who were already being treated for hypothyroidism with T4, suffered just as many symptoms related to the illness as those who had not begun any treatment for hypothyroidism in Table 2.

Again, my findings agree with those from the Hertoghe study. Obviously, treatment-using T4 is woefully lacking. Many of these patients' symptoms resolved after additional thyroid hormones were given.

I refer all inquiries that my office receives from Europe to the Belgian clinic:

Thierry Hertoghe
Brussels, Belgium
+ 32 2 736 68 68
www.hertoghe.eu
thhertoghe@gmx.net

Therese Hertoghe
Internal Medicine
Rue Pierre Delacroix, 23
1150 Brussels
00 32 2 463 03 00

Dr. Jacques Hertoghe and his colleagues introduced the T3-24 hour urine test in 1984. This test has proven itself to be the only reliable laboratory method that accurately measures thyroid function. Dr. Barnes' basal temperature test is the next best measure. Jerry Tennant M.D. has pioneered another method using blood tests that may prove to be effective as well.

# BASAL TEMPERATURE

DR. BARNES MEASURED the BMR as well as the basal temperature on every patient he treated. Numerous doctors had previously reported that a low basal temperature was almost always found in those suffering from hypothyroidism. During a tour of duty in World War II, Dr. Barnes studied 1,000 soldiers' temperatures. Prior to reveille, one thermometer would be placed in their mouth, one in their arm pit (axilla), and one in their rectum. If no sign of upper respiratory infection was present, he found that the oral temperature was within one tenth degree of the axillary temperature. The rectal temperature was eight tenths higher.

These findings conflict with standard medical textbooks that state the axillary temperature is one degree Fahrenheit lower than the oral temperature and two degrees Fahrenheit below the rectal temperature. However, no references are given to support their findings. Thyroid textbooks almost all state that the basal temperature test is invalid. Once again, absolutely no references are given. Dr. Barnes published his findings in his article entitled "Basal Temperature versus Basal Metabolism," which was published in the *Journal of the American Medical Association (JAMA)* in 1942.

After understanding Dr. Barnes research, I have utilized the basal temperature in all of the patients that I have treated for hypothyroidism.

Hypothyroid patients' temperatures are almost always below normal before they begin treatment. There are rare exceptions.

One of my former patients suffered emphysema. Her basal temperature was above normal because she had chronic lung infections, which are almost always present in emphysema patients. She had marked myxedema, a low hoarse voice, chronic pain, and anxiety. She also was over six feet tall. Many of her symptoms resolved after her dosage was slowly raised to 4 grains.

Just like the BMR, the basal temperature should be taken after a good night rest with no food, exercise, or excitement for 12 hours. Many patients who are hypothyroid may cover themselves with an excess number of blankets or quilts, sleep on a heated waterbed, wear long underwear, or layers of clothes to bed. All of these measures will falsely elevate the basal temperature. Women's temperatures fluctuate during their menstrual cycle, and their tests should be taken on the second and third days after menstrual flow starts. Babies and small children may be checked by rectal temperature for two minutes. I recommend a Geratherm thermometer.

To test your basal temperature, the thermometer is placed snugly in the armpit for 10 minutes before arising in the morning. Dr. Barnes found that temperature readings of 97.8 to 98.2° Fahrenheit (36.6 to 36.8° Celsius) were normal. Normal rectal temperatures are eight tenths degree higher, 98.6 to 99.2° Fahrenheit (37 to 37.3° Celsius).

During his lectures, Dr. Barnes stated that many of the adult patients he treated never attained normal basal body temperatures, even though they were given all the thyroid they were able to tolerate. Many of my adult patients' temperatures remain below normal even though their symptoms resolve.

The most important temperature readings are prior to being diagnosed with hypothyroidism. Once the diagnosis of hypothyroidism has been established and patients begin taking thyroid hormones, their basal temperatures will fluctuate for many months. The patients' temperatures will gradually increase as the thyroid dosage is raised.

# MY RECOMMENDATIONS ABOUT
# HOW TO BEGIN TREATMENT FOR HYPOTHYROIDISM
# TO PREVENT ALZHEIMER'S DISEASE

CARDIAC OUTPUT (BLOOD flow to the body from the heart) is often significantly decreased due to hypothyroidism. When beginning even small dosages of thyroid hormones, the heart muscle becomes stronger and beats more forcefully. If the coronary arteries supplying the heart are compromised by arterial sclerosis, the arteries may not be able to accommodate the increased blood flow, which is required. When the heart is deprived of the necessary blood flow, a heart attack may occur. Please follow my recommendations closely in order to minimize this danger.

Rule#1: Patients who have suffered a heart attack should not begin any thyroid medication for two months following a heart attack. I recommend such patients begin nitric oxide (NEO-40 www.neogenis.com) two or three times daily to help their arteries begin to recover. NEO-40 may be started immediately following a heart attack.

After 60 days, I recommend beginning 0.25 grains of thyroid every other day and slowly increasing the dosage by 0.25 grains every six or eight weeks until reaching a maximum of 2 grains daily. Dr. Barnes stated that anyone who has had a heart attack is much more sensitive to thyroid medication and should never take more than 2 grains of thyroid daily. My clinical experience is in complete agreement with Dr. Barnes' findings. However, almost every heart attack patient will require 2 grains of desiccated thyroid or the equivalent dosage of T4 and T3 if they have Hashimoto's (T4-76 mcg and T3-18 mcg).

Four of my patients suffered heart attacks within several months of beginning treatment with desiccated thyroid. I believe it is extremely prudent to begin thyroid hormones very slowly in anyone suspected of having coronary artery disease. Older patients who have had chronic dental problems and long-term hypothyroidism are at risk, especially if there is a family history of heart attack.

Rule #2: Patients who have high blood pressure must also begin thyroid medication cautiously. Too much thyroid medication initially will often further elevate their blood pressure and may cause serious problems. Begin 0.25 grains daily and increase the dosage by the same amount every six or eight weeks. If the blood pressure elevates, increase the dosage more gradually. Have the patients monitor their blood pressure at least twice a week and instruct them to stop their thyroid and report to their doctor if their pressure increases.

As they reach therapeutic levels of thyroid, their blood pressure often begins to drop. It may take one or two years for some patients to respond. Slowly wean patients off their blood pressure medications as pressure drops. It is often dangerous to stop blood pressure medications abruptly.

People who have advanced arterial disease may never be able to lower their blood pressure. Dr. Barnes reported such patients lived longer by taking thyroid versus similar patients who were not on thyroid.

Rule #3: A red flag for mild adrenal deficiency, iodine deficiency, thyroid antibodies, or environmental toxicity is a worsening of hypothyroid symptoms as the dosage is gradually increased. Stop or decrease the dosage of thyroid and address these problems should they occur. Less fatigue and symptomatic relief is the expected response.

If the basal temperature begins to decline, in addition to worsening symptoms, adrenal deficiency is almost always to blame. My first book includes chapters about adrenal deficiency, Hashimoto's, and Graves' disease.

Rule #4: There are always exceptions. Some patients have great difficulty tolerating any T4 and T3 preparations, including desiccated thyroid. My first book includes detailed recommendations for even the most difficult patients.

# GENERAL RECOMMENDATIONS

AFTER DOCTORS DISCOVERED how to successfully treat hypothyroidism in the late 1800s, there were no diagnostic tests to help them determine whether or not a patient suffered from hypothyroidism. Patients' medical histories, symptoms, and physical findings, combined with their doctors' awareness were the only means for making the diagnosis. A trial of thyroid hormones, leading to the resolution of the patient's symptoms and physical manifestations, was confirmation of a correct diagnosis. When combined with basal temperatures, I believe this method of treatment remains a viable option.

People who have below normal basal temperatures and suffer symptoms that are associated with hypothyroidism should begin a trial of thyroid hormones. Others with low basal temperatures and a family history that includes illnesses resulting from hypothyroidism, such as heart attacks or diabetes, should also begin a trial of thyroid hormones.

For most patients, I recommend 0.25 grains first thing in the morning on an empty stomach. Wait 30 minutes before eating because minerals block the absorption of the hormones. Increase the dosage monthly for adults. Younger patients who are relatively healthy may begin 0.5 grains and increase 0.5 grains monthly.

Estrogens protect the arteries of women who continue to have menstrual cycles. If these women do not have severe allergies or Hashimoto's disease, they may also increase their dosage by 0.5 grains every month.

As previously stated, the average adult dosage is about 3 grains every day. Dr. Barnes stated, "The bigger the beast, the bigger the bigger the bullet!" I have treated several 300 pound patients with 5 or 6 grains a day.

There are occasional patients who do not tolerate T3. Dr. Sonkin treated one family very successfully using large dosages of Synthroid (T4). A woman required 3 mg (about 30 times the amount that doctors currently recommend) and her son required 2.7 mg for restoration of their health. I asked Dr. Sonkin how he could possibly prescribe so much thyroid medication. His response was, "Because it took that much to wake them up!" The patients demonstrated no side effects and their symptoms markedly improved. Dr. Sonkin gradually increased their dosages and noted that the son had shown symptoms of thyrotoxicosis (an overdose) at 2.9 mg, which necessitated the slight decrease to 2.7 mg.

# TREATING CHILDREN AND TEENS

SMALL CHILDREN MAY begin 0.25 grains every other day. Compounding pharmacies can make liquid preparations for small children. I increase the dosage of thyroid every two months when treating children. Almost all the children that I have treated attained normal basal temperatures when they reached their correct dosage of thyroid. As they grow, their temperatures decline and their dosages are gradually increased. I insist that the children's parents monitor their child's heart rate and basal temperature every few weeks. The normal heart rate is much faster in children than adult heart rates and these rates are easily found on the Internet.

If a child's basal temperature is raised above normal, after beginning thyroid, immediately stop the thyroid until the temperature returns to the normal range. Begin a lower dosage of thyroid. Hyperthermia (elevated basal temperature above normal) indicates hyperthyroidism and can cause severe problems including death. Of course, this does not apply if the child is ill and has a fever.

A heart rate above normal (when resting) is a strong indication that the patient is not tolerating the thyroid hormones. Additional symptoms of intolerance include palpitations, shortness of breath, chest pain, increased fatigue, increased anxiety, increased insomnia, trembling hands, and increased joint and muscle pain.

Many of the teenagers I have treated eventually required between 2 and 3 grains a day, depending upon their size. Many teens are the size of adults and require similar dosages.

# TREATMENT FOR HASHIMOTO'S AND GRAVES' DISEASE

THE INCIDENCE OF autoimmune thyroid disease called Hashimoto's thyroiditis is rapidly increasing in America. Hashimoto's disease means your immune system is attacking your own thyroid gland. A recent study indicated that about 5% of Americans might be affected.

None of Dr. Barnes' four books mentioned Hashimoto's thyroiditis. It was very rare at that time. Near the end of his recorded lecture, Dr. Barnes answered questions from the doctors who were in attendance. When asked about Hashimoto's, Dr. Barnes stated that you must use the synthetic hormones if the patent has Hashimoto's. The synthetic hormones are levothyroxine or L-thyroxin (T4) and Triiodothyronine (T3). The generic name for T3 is liothyronine and the brand name is Cytomel®.

Why would Dr. Barnes recommend synthetic hormones? Desiccated porcine (pig) thyroid is almost identical to our own thyroid gland. Pigs are genetically quite similar to humans. If the body is attacking the thyroid gland, adding more glandular thyroid is like adding fuel to the fire. However, there are a small number of patients who feel much better when taking desiccated thyroid, in spite of the fact that they have Hashimoto's disease.

The tests to determine if you have Hashimoto's are called tissue peroxidase antibodies (TPO antibodies) and thyroglobulin antibodies. If you are found to have Hashimoto's and your basal temperature is below normal, I recommend taking a combination of T4 and T3 thyroid hormones.

*Hashimoto's and non-Hashimoto's patients require similar dosages; adults and children alike.*

Almost all of my patients who have had Graves' disease have already had chemical destruction or surgical removal of their thyroid glands. Patients with a history of Graves' usually require synthetic T4 and T3 in order to restore their health.

A new book authored by Mary Shomon entitled *Living Well with Graves' Disease and Hyperthyroidism* offers more conservative treatments to reverse Graves' disease. Additional information is available on a growing number of Web sites including aboutthyroid.com, stopthethyroidmadness.com, and brodabarnes.org.

I always check for thyroid antibodies after chemical destruction or removal of the thyroid gland. In spite of the fact that the thyroid gland has been destroyed or removed, patients with a history of autoimmune thyroid illnesses often have high levels of thyroid antibodies.

Depending upon whether or not patients have thyroid antibodies usually dictates whether they will require T4 and T3 versus desiccated thyroid. I have had two average-sized adult patients who required 6 grains of thyroid to feel well after removal of their thyroid gland. I gradually increased their dosages over many months.

Patients who have autoimmune thyroid illnesses often suffer from severe allergies. I recommend that these patients seek help from environmental medicine physicians. Doctors belonging to the American Academy of Environmental Medicine (aaemonline.com) are able to diagnose and successfully treat severe food and environmental allergies much more effectively than other allergists.

# CONVERSION RATIOS OF THYROID HORMONES

DESICCATED THYROID CONTAINS glandular thyroid and is measured in milligrams. One grain of desiccated thyroid weighs about 65 mg and contains 38 micrograms of T4 and 9 micrograms of T3. Armour thyroid dosages are slightly different because they reference 1 grain = 60 mg. However, the stated amounts of T4 and T3 are the same (T4-38 mcg and T3-9 mcg).

Synthetic T4 and T3 are bio-identical synthetic hormones that are derived from sugar beets. T4 and T3 are measured in micrograms.

Pharmacies must use fillers to accurately measure microgram dosages. Many of my patients who had autoimmune thyroid illnesses became allergic to the most common filler, which is named methylcellulose. It is derived from pine and is allergenic. I recommend using potato starch, acidophilus, or Avicel® for fillers because they less allergenic. I have found that calcium carbonate also works well, in spite of the fact that calcium is supposed to block absorption of thyroid hormones.

**Conversion of grains to desiccated thyroid:**
**1 grain = T4-38 mcg and T3-9 mcg**
**0.25 grains = T4-9.5 mcg and T3-2.25 mcg**
**2 grains = T4-76 mcg and T3-18 mcg**
**3 grains = T4-114 mcg and T3-27 mcg.**

A number of countries, including Brazil, have never had access to desiccated thyroid. A doctor from Brazil is a patient of mine. He read my first book and came to my clinic in Arizona. His health has improved since he began desiccated thyroid.

# TOXIC SOUP

## UMBILICAL CORD BLOOD STUDY

A 2004 U.S. study by the Environmental Working Group (EWG) revealed that pregnant women's umbilical cord blood is contaminated with an average of 200 industrial chemicals and pollutants. Of the 287 chemicals detected, 180 are known to cause cancer in humans or animals, 217 are toxic to the brain and nervous system, and 208 cause birth defects or abnormal development in animals.

In 2009, EWG repeated the study and found an average of 232 chemicals in umbilical cord blood. If you do the math, most of these toxins cause all three problems. These are noxious poisons.

What we do to our planet, we do to ourselves.

In addition to being poisonous, a majority of these toxins adversely affect most of our hormones including the thyroid. A wonderful book on this subject is *Our Stolen Future*. The Web site (ourstolenfuture.org) is a great resource about how to protect yourself and your children from toxins that are adversely affecting our hormones.

If you have any of the conditions listed throughout this book, you should seek help from a physician who understands how to properly diagnose and treat hypothyroidism.

# CASE STUDIES

## MYXEDEMA: THE TELLTALE SIGN OF HYPOTHYROIDISM

In 1878, Dr. William Ord performed an autopsy on a middle-aged woman who succumbed to hypothyroidism. Upon cutting into her skin, he saw tissues that were thickened and boggy. The tissues appeared to be waterlogged, but no water seeped from his incisions. Dr. Ord realized this disease was unique and previously unrecognized.

Dr. Ord summoned a leading chemist named Halleburton to help identify the substance causing the swelling. What they found was an abnormally large accumulation of mucin. Mucin is a normal constituent of our tissues. It is a jelly-like material that spontaneously accumulates in hypothyroidism. Mucin grabs onto water and causes swelling. Dr. Halleburton found 50 times the normal amount of mucin in the woman's skin. Her other tissues also contained excess mucin.

The doctors coined the term "myxedema". "Myx" is the Greek word for mucin and "edema" means swelling. "Myxedema" was adopted as the medical term for hypothyroidism.

The edema or swelling associated with hypothyroidism usually begins around the face, particularly above or below the eyes and along the jaw line. However, the skin on the side of the upper arms may be thickened early in the course of the disease. The swelling associated with hypothyroidism is firm and will eventually spread throughout our body's connective tissues.

One of the many functions of connective tissue is to help hold our bodies' organs and structures together. Connective tissue lines our blood vessels, nervous system, muscles, mucous membranes (such as the sinuses), the gut, as well as each and every cell in our glands and organs. Abnormal accumulation of mucin in these tissues causes swelling and significantly impairs normal function.

This type of swelling is unique to hypothyroidism. Medical textbooks about hypothyroidism state that myxedema is thyroprival (pertaining to or characterized by hypothyroidism) and pathognomonic (specifically distinctive and diagnostic). Translation: if the thickened skin or myxedema is present, you have hypothyroidism.

Do you have myxedema? As I stated, aside from the face, one of the first places affected are the lateral upper arms. Try to pinch the skin as demonstrated in the picture. The swollen skin on this patient's arm, as well as the puffiness in her hand, is a classic demonstration of myxedema.

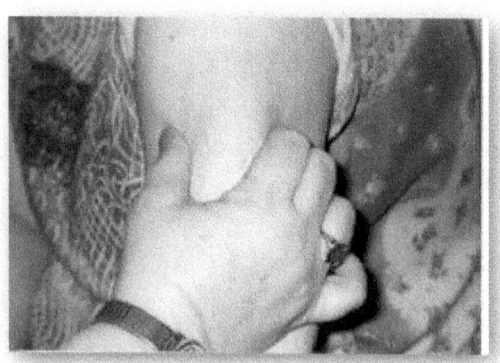

**Marked Myxedema**

Early 20th century literature about hypothyroidism included photographs that demonstrated myxedema before and after treatment. The puffiness or myxedema in the patients' faces and hands remarkably improved.[2]

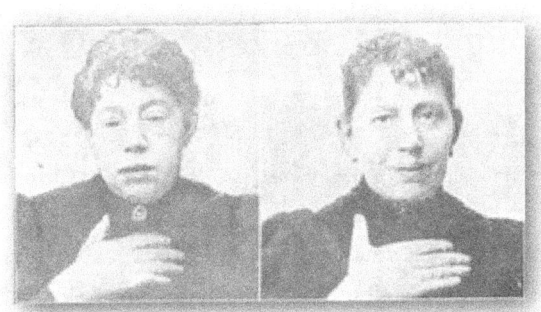

Before treatment          After treatment

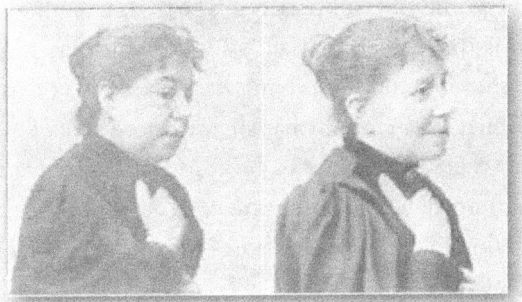

Before treatment          After treatment

Source: Hertoghe E. *The Practitioner.* Jan 1915; Vol XCIV, No 1:26-93.

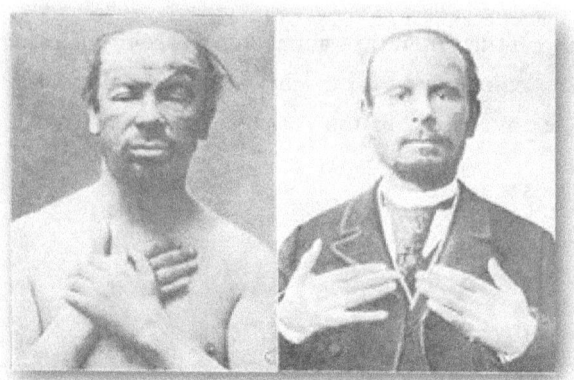

Source: Hertoghe E. *The Practitioner.* Jan 1915; Vol XCIV, No 1:26-93.

It is important that you pinch in the same area. Next, try to lift the skin off the underlying tissue on your arm. Normal skin is relatively thin, and you may easily lift it with your thumb and index finger. I have examined a number of patients whose skin is almost impossible to lift. This is due to the marked swelling and glue-like infiltration of mucin in the skin and underlying tissues that result from hypothyroidism. Women's skin usually has slightly more subcutaneous fat than men. Hence, their skin tends to be thicker. There are many different degrees of myxedema. I use *marked, moderate,* and *mild* to describe them. The following picture illustrates normal skin thickness.

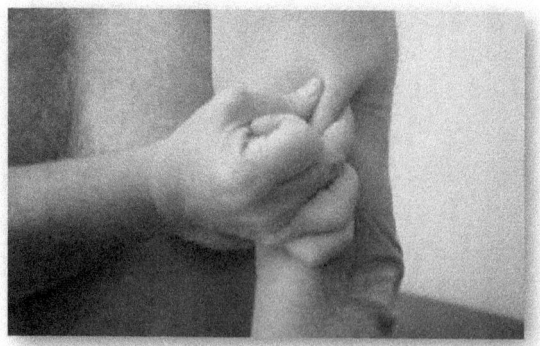

*Normal Skin Thickness of the Upper Lateral Arm*

Unfortunately, even if your skin is of normal thickness, you may still have the hypothyroidism. It is only one of many signs of this disease.

Today's doctors are not taught to examine for thickened skin or other physical manifestations of the illness. Sophisticated thyroid blood tests are purported to be the sole means for making the diagnosis of hypo-thyroidism. These tests have replaced the patients' medical histories, complaints, and physical findings upon which the diagnosis was largely based for over half a century before the advent of blood tests.

I raised the ire of many physicians by remarking on the marked myx-edema present in their patients. This diagnostic clinical finding has been forgotten, usurped by the almighty thyroid blood tests.

One patient of mine, a 55 year-old suffering from hypo-thyroidism, returned to his primary care doctor for confirmation of my diagnosis. The patient was obese, suffering chronic pain, fatigue, dry skin, high blood pressure, a slightly irregular heartbeat, and sleep apnea. The skin on his upper arms and the front of his thighs was quite thickened with myxedema. The primary care doctor told the patient the thickened skin was due to his obesity. The patient and his wife were concerned with the conflicting views. Fortunately, he finally decided to follow my advice.

After many months of treatment for hypothyroidism, his chronic fatigue vastly improved, his heartbeat normalized, high blood pressure resolved, and the thickness of his skin normalized. The myxedema had disappeared. I told the patient to tell his primary care doctor that his skin had been on a crash diet. Pictures of his skin one year after begin-ning thyroid hormones are shown on the next page.

Modern medical textbooks about hypothyroidism prominently mention its effect on the heart. Cardiac output (blood flow from the heart to the rest of the body) is often reduced to one half the normal value. However, most CHF patients who suffer hypothyroidism are not identified because the thyroid hormone blood tests are missing the vast majority of patients suffering from the illness. When patients are identified with hypothyroidism, the dosages that doctors have been taught to use for the last 40 years are ineffectual and do not resolve congestive heart failure.

The last medical textbook that contained "before treatment" and "after treatment" photographs was published in 1957. Its distinguished authors were Dr. Lisser, President of the American Endocrine Society, and Dr. Escamilla, both of whom spent their careers at the University of California Endocrinology Clinic in San Francisco.

The following photographs and case study are from Dr. Escamilla's and Dr. Lisser's 1957 textbook. They represent a remarkable illustration of how wrong the treatment for hypothyroidism has become.

# THE MEDICAL SCHOOL MODEL

IN THE LATE 1980s, when I was in medical school, I saw several patients with this constellation of symptoms. Medical students were taught to remove the fluid from patients' abdomens (peritoneal cavity) with a large needle. We would prescribe medications for the heart and were instructed to use laxatives and enemas in order to relieve severe constipation.

Since I began proper treatment for hypothyroidism, none of my patients have ever developed congestive heart failure.

Unfortunately, several of my colleagues and I have found that it is extremely difficult to successfully treat patients with severe congestive heart failure. The old adage that an ounce of prevention is worth a pound of cure could not be more true.

# REFERENCES

Barnes BO. Thyroid Therapy I, II, III (Audio Tapes) Copies available through The Broda O. Barnes M.D. Research Foundation (www.brodabarnes.org).

Wallace D. Mitochondrial DNA in aging and disease. Scientific American. August 1997.

Freidman E, Cain W. The New Testosterone Treatment: How You and Your Doctor Can Fight Breast Cancer, Prostate Cancer, and Alzheimer's. Prometheus Books. 2013.

FN Peterson / Friedman

Freidman E, Cain W. The New Testosterone Treatment: How You and Your Doctor Can Fight Breast Cancer, Prostate Cancer, and Alzheimer's. Prometheus Books. 2013.

*Weston Price Foundation westonprice.org/know-your-fats*

Unpublished material, received via personal communication from Carol Petersen RPh, CNP, Marketing Liaison, Women's International Pharmacy / Pet Health Pharmacy. Madison, WI. www.womensinternational.com

Unpublished material, received via personal communication from Cathy Stuart, Executive Director, Arizona Naturopathic Medical Association, Goodyear, AZ. www.aznma.org

Pacholok S, Stuart J; Could It Be B12-An Epidemic of Misdiagnoses, Quill Driver Books, 2005

Brownstein D. Vitamin B12 for Health, ISBN:978-0-9660882-9-8. Medical Alternatives Press, 4173 Fieldbrook, Wes Bloomfield, MI. 2012.

Zandi PP, Carlson MC, Plassman BL, et al. Hormone replacement therapy and incidence of Alzheimer disease in older women: The Cache County Study. JAMA. 2002 Nov 6;288(17):2123-2129.

Hargrove JT, Osteen KG. An alternative method of hormone replacement therapy
The healthimpact.com/2012/coconutoil-and-alzheimer's

Boyle R. The report that shocked the President. Sports Illustrated. July 1955.

Kraus H, Marcus NJ. Technological advance amidst humanistic decline: Ignoring muscle evaluation and treatment in the modern age of medicine. Journal of Back and Musculoskeletal Rehabilitation. 1997; 8(2):83-85.

Hill RB, Anderson RE. The recent history of the autopsy. Archives Pathology Lab Med: Historical Perspective. 1996; 120:702-712.

McPhee S. The autopsy: An antidote to misdiagnosis. Medicine. 1996; 75(1):41-43.

Ross R. Mechanisms of Disease—Atherosclerosis—An inflammatory disease. New England Journal of Medicine. 1999; 340(2):115-123.

Strong JP, McGill HC. The pediatric aspects of atherosclerosis. Journal Atherosclerosis Research. 1969; 9:251.

Ord WM. On myoxoedema, a term proposed to be applied to an essential condition in the cretinoid infection occasionally observed in middle- aged women. Trans Med-Churg Society London. 1877-1878; 60-1:57-78.

Barnes BO., Ratzenhofer M, Gisi R. The role of natural consequences in the changing death patterns. Journal American of the American Geriatrics Society. 1974; 22:176.

Campbell RE., Hughes FA. The development of bronchogenic carcinoma in patients with pulmonary tuberculosis. J Thorac Cardiovasc Surgery. 1960; 40:89-101.

Barnes BO. Heart Attack Rareness in Thyroid–Treated Patients. Springfield, IL: Charles C. Thomas. 1972.

Barnes BO. Solved: The Riddle of Heart Attacks. Trumbull, CT: The Broda O. Barnes M.D. Research Foundation. 1976.

Congress of the European Society of Cardiology, Stockholm Sweden. January 2002.

Espinola-Klein C, Rupprecht HJ, Blankenberg S, Bickel C, Kopp H, Rippin G, et al. Impact of infectious burden on extent and long-term prognosis of atherosclerosis. Circulation. 2002; 105(1):15-21.

Braunwald E. Shattuck lecture—cardiovascular medicine at the turn of the millennium: Triumphs, concerns and opportunities. New England Journal of Medicine. 1997; 337(19):1360-1369.
http://www.ncbi.nlm.nih.gov/pubmed/22775208

Dr. Higginson I. Pepler WJ: Fat intake, serum cholesterol concentration, and atherosclerosis in the South African Bantu. Part II. Atherosclerosis and coronary artery disease. Journal ClinicalInvestigation 33: *1366, 1954*

www.ingramcontent.com/pod-product-compliance
Lightning Source LLC
Chambersburg PA
CBHW070253190526
45169CB00001B/392